P9-CDX-514

BIRTH
WITHOUT
FEAR

BIRTH WITHOUT FEAR

January Harshe

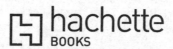

hachette
BOOKS

NEW YORK   BOSTON

LONDON PUBLIC LIBRARY

This book is intended to provide helpful and informative material. It is not intended to diagnose, treat, cure, or prevent any health problem or condition, nor is intended to replace the advice of a physician. No action should be taken solely on the contents of this book. Always consult your physician or qualified health care provider on any matters regarding your health and before adopting any suggestions in this book or drawing inferences from it.

Copyright © 2019 by January Harshe

Cover design by Amanda Kain
Illustration © baldygran/Shutterstock
Cover copyright © 2019 by Hachette Book Group, Inc.

Hachette Book Group supports the right to free expression and the value of copyright. The purpose of copyright is to encourage writers and artists to produce the creative works that enrich our culture.

The scanning, uploading, and distribution of this book without permission is a theft of the author's intellectual property. If you would like permission to use material from the book (other than for review purposes), please contact permissions@hbgusa.com. Thank you for your support of the author's rights.

Hachette Books
Hachette Book Group
1290 Avenue of the Americas
New York, NY 10104
hachettebooks.com
twitter.com/hachettebooks

First Edition: March 2019

Hachette Books is a division of Hachette Book Group, Inc.
The Hachette Books name and logo are trademarks of Hachette Book Group, Inc.

The publisher is not responsible for websites (or their content) that are not owned by the publisher.

The Hachette Speakers Bureau provides a wide range of authors for speaking events. To find out more, go to www.hachettespeakersbureau.com or call (866) 376-6591.

Library of Congress Cataloging-in-Publication Data

Names: Harshe, January, author.
Title: Birth without fear / by January Harshe.
Description: First edition. | New York, NY: Hachette Books, [2019] | Includes
    bibliographical references and index.
Identifiers: LCCN 2018020001| ISBN 9780316515610 (trade paperback) | ISBN
    9780316515597 (ebook)
Subjects: LCSH: Pregnancy—Popular works. | Childbirth—Popular works. | Pregnant
    women—Health and hygiene—Popular works. | Puerperium—Popular works.
Classification: LCC RG525 .H358 2019 | DDC 618.2—dc23
LC record available at https://lccn.loc.gov/2018020001

ISBNs: 978-0-316-51561-0 (trade paperback), 978-0-316-51559-7 (ebook)

Printed in the United States of America

LSC-C

10 9 8 7 6 5 4 3 2

To my six babies. None of this would be possible without you.

Contents

Introduction

Honesty in womanhood and motherhood is what
creates a sisterhood.

A birth without fear.

That was the answer.

It was an answer that came to me during nap time. Not *my* nap time, of course. As a mother of four, my youngest just eleven months old, I wasn't sleeping very much. In fact, I was sleeping so little that I probably should have been trying to catch a few moments of rest as I lay side by side with my snoozing baby girl one late morning in May. Instead my mind was at work.

"But they let you?" I remembered a friend's response when I told her about my most recent birth experience. I was a plus-size, post-due-date, VBAC (vaginal birth after cesarean) birthing mama, and pretty much everyone I told about my home birth replied with disbelief. "I had to have *x, y, and z,*" they all seemed to say. "Otherwise they wouldn't have allowed it." What struck me most about these conversations was how all of the power was with some external authority, not with the mother. *Let* you? *Allow? Had to have?*

These words smacked hard against the reality of my recent drug-free home birth experience. I could only describe my labor this time around as peaceful, healing, and even euphoric. My husband, Brandon, described it as the best day of his life.

But I also understood the disbelief my friends and family

expressed, for I too had experienced powerlessness during birth. With my first child, a planned birthing center birth with midwives turned into a scheduled cesarean with a high-risk OB/GYN; with my second, a planned VBAC at home, fifty-two hours of labor turned into an emergency cesarean. My third was another planned home birth; this time a VBA2C (vaginal birth after two cesareans) turned into a hospital birth characterized by disrespect, violation, and bullying from the doctor and nurse-midwife.

I wondered what made this sweet baby's birth so different from the older three.

The answer came to me in an unexpected instant: Fear was not a factor.

With pregnancy number four, my determination and confidence in my body prevailed. I knew my body could birth a baby the way millions of women had birthed babies before me, and I knew the only person who knew I could do it was me. I had trust and faith in myself and I refused to let all those noisy, anxious doubts and fears disrupt that for me.

You see, in the hospital I always found myself strapped to machines for the nurses and anesthesiologists to monitor while OB/GYNs prepped for cesareans. Hospital billing staff came and went with form after form after form for me to sign. The fear that something *might* go wrong or, with a vital sign slightly off the average, that something *was* going wrong guided every decision. If my newborn was not a certain weight or nursing at specific intervals or in this percentile or that percentile, the pediatricians on call panicked. Once home, I felt shell-shocked, out of touch with my body and my voice, and now with the additional task of caring for a brand-new, fragile baby after such frantic experiences.

As my fourth baby lay fast asleep next to me that day, her two fingers acting as a pacifier, I thought back to the moments and hours following this cuddlebug's birth: holding her for many ecstatic moments before giving her my breast; nursing her for a short time as I examined her precious rolls and wrinkles; falling asleep with her in my arms; waking up and handing her to Brandon so I could clean myself up and put on clothes; going to the couch, joyously taking the baby back in my arms to nurse her again; the kids waking up and celebrating the birth of their new sister with ear-to-ear grins—everything just as I had visualized it years earlier when I was pregnant with my first child.

Perfect.

Later that day, as Brandon and I did lots of processing about this baby's peaceful birth, the Birth Without Fear community was born. We started by creating a Facebook page. At the time it seemed to be what everyone was doing and we wanted a way to reach as many women as possible as fast as possible. It seemed more effective than shouting from a bullhorn.

We decided on the name Birth Without Fear to celebrate the kinds of birth experiences that empowered moms and families. At the same time, we worried the assumption of fear might be too negative—I knew other women who experienced fear in childbirth, as I did with my first three children, but I didn't know how far it reached beyond my community. How many others struggled with a lack of good information, as I did? How many had experiences where they felt disrespected or judged? Seven years and more than half a million followers later, it is clear we hit a nerve.

I did not have my name attached to Birth Without Fear at first. It was an anonymous place for me to share a lot of information about pregnancy and birth options. So many women I talked to in my own life did not feel they were allowed to have a say in how they birthed. They didn't realize there were options and alternative approaches; or, if they did, they had no clue how to get their hands on the information. There was no place for us to collectively come together as women to share our experiences and information, and to support one another. After a few months, women who joined our community asked to share their own stories, and that is how the blog and website began.

I created Birth Without Fear as a way to offer information and support so that women could have more experiences like those I had with my fourth child: peaceful, empowering births where fear didn't have to be the motivating factor. I wanted a platform from which I could stand up for women who opted not to have the standard hospital birth. It was a message of strength and empowerment for anyone wanting to walk the lesser-known path. Within a few short months, Birth Without Fear accumulated tens of thousands of followers, and I could see that it wasn't just a website, but a movement for women seeking information and affirmation. A place where they could find different, more supportive answers than they were getting from their birth care providers. A voice for us all both collectively and individually.

But soon I started to wonder about the voice I had given to Birth Without Fear. Yes, it was empowering. Yes, it was inspirational. Yes, it was feisty. But something was missing. I knew there was no mistaking that my second and third births ended in last-minute disappointment and trauma and that my home birth was a healing experience for myself and Brandon. However, the more I reflected, I realized I had only been telling part of my birth story. My first birth experience—a scheduled cesarean with an OB/GYN—had been a positive, even peaceful event in its own right.

My high-risk OB/GYN was calm, respectful, and gave me the opportunity to voice my thoughts and concerns. *Together* we decided that a cesarean at 39½ weeks was the best decision for me and my baby. When I presented him with a specific, gentle cesarean birth plan (not a label or movement at the time) that I wanted followed in detail for the actual birth and postpartum stay, the doctor gladly signed off on it, seeing to it that my every wish was respected. The birth itself was smooth and flawless. My baby was the first ever in that hospital not to go to the nursery following a cesarean birth. The nurses were kind and helpful. The pediatrician was considerate of my wishes. Family and friends made up for the terrible hospital food with a steady procession of meals that Brandon's appetite more than appreciated.

Reflecting on this experience reminded me that birth was far from a black-or-white thing, where drug-free home births are "good" and hospital births with interventions are "bad." There are so many shades of gray. Indeed, from my own life I knew that a more traditional hospital birth—including a C-section—*could* be an extremely positive experience, full of options, support, and respect. If I wanted to be true to myself and my community, I needed to step down from my soapbox (well, most of the time) and meet women and families with complete honesty. Only then could they meet me and each other in the same authentic, loving spirit. Only then could I help them have births without fear in any situation.

This crystallized the Birth Without Fear way as a movement for *all* women and birthing people. A community of grace and understanding, a place where women choosing C-sections and vaginal births, women who feel more comfortable in a hospital instead of a birthing center, women who feel more comfortable at home than in a hospital, women choosing to feed their babies formula instead of breastfeeding, women choosing to exclusively breastfeed beyond the societal norms, women from small towns and those in big cities, homeschooling and corporate mamas, lesbian, bisexual, queer, and trans birthing people, women of color, and every variation of mother in between can all come together with support and respect taking the place of competition and judgment.

Today the Birth Without Fear community is much more than a Facebook page. It's a community a million strong that reaches from the United States to Australia and many places in between. From that one social media group we have sprouted a range of communities encompassing all aspects of the parenting journey with groups such as Take Back Postpartum, Breastfeed Without Fear, Find Your Village, and Don't Forget Dads. And we've moved out of cyberspace and into in-person gatherings—I travel the world hosting Birth Without Fear and Find Your Village events where I get to snuggle lots of your sweet babies and hold your hands as you share your stories.

Brandon helps me run the Birth Without Fear blog, serves as webmaster and blog editor, and is as involved in the decision-making process and evolution of Birth Without Fear and the Birth Without Fear events as he was on that first day when our fourth child was born and we decided to start a Facebook page. We also now have a podcast, *The Harshē Podcast*, which Brandon co-hosts with me and serves as the (sometimes inappropriate) comic relief.

Whenever possible—and it's admittedly hard with six kids—Brandon joins me as a speaker at Birth Without Fear events, where he shares what he's learned (and is learning) as a father of six and as my central support person through pregnancies, loss, births, and postpartum.

They say practice makes perfect, and that we learn through our experiences. Through repeated pregnancies and births I grew more and more confident in my body and my voice, and I also grew more aware of the realities of birth in the United States. Given an unlimited number of births (or, in my case, six), you'd probably make the same connections I did by baby number four—that it matters less how your baby is born and more how you are treated during your labor, and that this guiding principle ripples out beyond birth to include pregnancy, postpartum, parenting, and, hell, even your whole life. Our lives don't have to look the same, just as our bodies, our pregnancies, and our families don't have to look the same, but it matters that our experience of the journey is respected, that we have options, and that we have the support we need.

Without multiple experiences with which to compare and explore the ins and outs of birth, all we have is each other's stories to fill in those gaps of experience. Even with my own widely varying experiences, I *still* needed a village of support. No matter how much we may be conditioned to believe that life is a series of stages we accomplish either successfully or not and then move onto the next, it is in fact a much messier, ongoing, nonlinear journey. Our best resource to help us keep showing up to our lives is each other.

Most women and families don't have an unlimited number of births to figure things out. Many of us struggle to find a strong village of support. Far too often we make decisions that stem from the subconscious belief that we have to listen to authority, that our feelings aren't valid, or that it's our responsibility to take care of others more than ourselves. Care providers—everyone from OBs and midwives to lactation consultants and therapists—can so easily confirm our feelings of powerlessness by not including us in their recommendations and decisions. Pop culture and social media swoop in to offer us so many "right" ways to live, birth, and parent that our voices and our individuality can get more lost to us every time we refresh our newsfeeds. At any stage of our lives we can learn (and relearn) how to be advocates for ourselves and each other in the face of so many other influences.

I hear so many stories of fear from the Birth Without Fear community: fear of all the unknowns in fertility, pregnancy, birth, and parenting; fear of whether or not they can get pregnant or that their "advanced maternal age" will cause complications; fear that they'll go into labor when their OB/GYN is not on call and that their birth plans will go out the window; fear of bringing previous traumatic experiences with one baby into a next pregnancy, whether it's an episiotomy or a baby born with heart defects that went undetected; fear that they're not going to be able to handle the pain or the sleep deprivation; fear of being bullied into another C-section when trying for a VBAC; fear of making it past their due date or not making it to their due date, and the cascade of interventions that will surely follow. There is just too much fear associated with pregnancy, birth, and postpartum—understandably so—and not nearly enough support.

The journey for a birth without fear (and a pregnancy without fear, and a postpartum without fear, and a life without fear, etc.) doesn't mean that you have no fear—it means having the courage to name and acknowledge your fears so that they no longer have so much power over you. In this book, I'm not going to tell you not to feel ashamed or scared or hurt anymore because I know that those feelings are valid and real. But I am going to help you name the things that feel limiting and empower you to find more options. I'll encourage you to speak your own truths and listen to other women with grace and compassion, for it is this honesty that creates a sisterhood, a village, so that we know we are not alone.

These days "self-care" is such a loaded term. It's so popular and mainstream at the moment that we all feel we *should* be doing it, but most of us really have no clue what it is or how to apply it to our lives. We're made to think it means taking a warm bath filled with Instagram-able rose petals, but in reality it means doing the work, day in and day out, of finding the woman beyond the wife, partner, and mother.

But in order to do that work, we need to practice being honest with ourselves and with others. We need to keep it real, because when you use your voice you not only empower yourself but other women who hear you. It gives them power to use their voice as well. Our stories and experiences are valuable wisdom. It's about empowerment, inspiration, support, healing, solidarity, and validation—from trying to conceive, to pregnancy, and from birth to postpartum and beyond.

Unlike some pregnancy books that tell you what to expect, as if it were that easy to distill the beautiful diversity of birth into a singular narrative, this book is about creating the space for birth narratives that empower all women, all bodies, and all families to get the most out of their journeys.

In the pages that follow I'll glean the wisdom of the community to resist the one-size-fits-all, fear-based medical model of birth, but not so that in its place I just create another singular version of "normal." Instead, my goal is to expand the notion of birth into as many variations as there are bodies, babies, and families. It's a way for us to hold on to our individuality without losing the benefits of the medical knowledge. I'll help all mothers and families assess their normal—as I often say of my own parenting style: "Some days it's all organic raw vegan. Other days it's Oreos and Coke. That's my kind of balance." I'm here to help you get in touch with *your* power and possibility, to find the balance that feels right for you.

Each chapter is filled to the brim with information empowering you to make the best decisions for your life, and it's also filled with stories: stories from my six different pregnancies, birth, and postpartum experiences; from Brandon's experiences; and from the diverse and beautiful Birth Without Fear community. Why? Because this book does more than simply give you information—it *creates* a village for you, one that validates and embraces all the variations of normal. I invite you to gather round. I also encourage you to be inspired by these stories to claim your own pregnancy, birth, and postpartum stories. This is a revolutionary community where women and partners can gather, be heard, and be held. It's a space free of judgment, where we can all take a deep breath and really listen. It's a commitment to hold each other in joy, stress, and even grief and anger.

This book is divided into three sections: pregnancy, birth, and postpartum. However, although the book starts with pregnancy and ends in postpartum, as this seems the most logical, linear time line to follow, we acknowledge that our journeys are never that neat, fixed, or finite. Sure, sometimes a positive over-the-counter pregnancy test is the first step on a woman's birth journey, but another woman could just as easily talk about the first time she looked into her future husband's eyes, or even a longing for motherhood she had as a young girl playing with dolls, as the beginning of her baby journey—and others may recount months and months spent at fertility clinics. And so beginnings are not as standardized as they may seem.

On the other end of things, there are plenty of "experts" defining postpartum for women. Six weeks, some say. Twelve weeks, according to others. These recommendations stigmatize and shame the many women for whom postpartum lasts much longer. This book passionately demands a shift in that narrative. We are changing the conversation. Right now. In reality, postpartum can last more like two years—or however long it takes to go through adjustments and struggles as we work through changes and find a new normal.

Of course, there are some clearly defined stages of pregnancy, birth, and child development, but there is also a beautiful and dynamic range of normal within those stages that must be acknowledged if we are to empower women in their parenting journeys. Just as labor has its own time and rhythms, this book creates movement within the linear chapter time line in order to hold space for readers to find themselves on their own terms. We're all on our own journeys and we all take our own time. One size does not fit all; in celebrating our individuality we can find true solidarity, healing, and validation.

Partners and spouses are featured in every chapter of this book in Brandon's "Partner Point of View" sections, because their empowerment and support matters, too. There is a stigma against active fatherhood, or partners who want to be helpful but don't really know what to do (and don't have role models they can turn to). They, too, deal with social and media misrepresentation and stigmas. Just as this book creates a community for women, it will also be a voice for men and all kinds of partners by addressing the range of feelings they, too, can have and the many ways they can join in the parenthood journey.

As I wrote this book, I found myself straining to imagine every possibility you might face so that I could help prevent any hurt or trauma in your pregnancy, birth, and postpartum journey. I'd be up late at night worrying and wondering and trying to plan for every outcome. It just felt so overwhelming and impossible. In fact, I realized, it *is* impossible. There's no way I could keep every stress, hurt, or challenge from you.

More than that, though, I came to the understanding that I wouldn't even want to keep you from having the growth on your journey that you're supposed to have. I remembered that if I hadn't had my traumatic birth experiences and then fought for myself to have healing birth experiences I would never have started *Birth Without Fear* in the first place and wouldn't have had the honor of writing this book at all. My fight to speak up for myself and my babies made me who I am. Those experiences hurt; they were painful and difficult and they tested me to my very bones. But they were important for me. And they are important for all of us—the hard ones and the good ones, they're all important.

I can't take or keep those bad experiences from you, and it wouldn't be right for me to do so anyway because they're your experiences to learn and grow from. But I can walk next to you, side by side, as you go on your journey. Not in front to lead you, or behind to follow, but beside you to hold your hand so that you know you're not alone. I want to empower you to process, heal, and go through your journey in your own way. That solidarity and love are the heart of this book. Acceptance and empowerment are front and center.

If you are thinking about getting pregnant or you are pregnant, this book is for you. If you are a new mother, this book is for you. If you are a husband or partner, this book is for you. If you are a birth care provider, this book is for you.

Simply put, if you are a human being, this book is for you.

PART ONE

· ·

Empowered Pregnancy

Love yourself enough to get the care you deserve.

In the following chapters I'll hold space for you, your variations of normal, and your pregnancy from your first trimester to your last. Every pregnancy is different. Even if you've already had children, every pregnancy is unique. Don't skip these chapters. Take the time to hear the encouragement, support, and love. Whether you're a first-time mom or mother of many, these chapters are going to remind you of the power you already have within you. Being pregnant can be mentally and physically challenging. Even if you have a simple or easy pregnancy. It becomes your whole world. But the world around you doesn't stop being the way that it is. The only person you can count on to validate that is you. Make sure you're loving and honoring yourself first and then it expands out from there to your partner, spouse, friends, family, and birth team.

I'm not going to tell you what to expect during your pregnancy. This is not a week-by-week guide. No one can tell you exactly how to feel or how this pregnancy is going to go. It's impossible. Instead I want to give you the wisdom of your mom, aunts, and sisters that you never had. I'm bringing together thousands of women's voices and experiences and sharing their wisdom with you, women who've witnessed each other as women—not the media's version of us, or the medical narrative of us—but our own and each other's power. You're holding the collective voice of thousands of women in your hands.

Chapter 1

Variations of Normal:
First Trimester Without Fear

....

Y ou are unique. You are not like any other pregnant woman before you, currently, or to come. Even your previous pregnancies, if you've had them, are different from this one. There is such a constellation of things that make you *you* and your pregnancy *your pregnancy*—from geography to the idiosyncrasies of your body. Take refuge in the experiences of others when they are a source of comfort, solidarity, and useful information, with the knowledge that every single pregnant person—and her baby—is unique.

I'm not here to tell you that you'll feel this or that. I'm here to offer you this healing perspective: everything you feel is a variation of normal. You may experience all the things you see on television, or read online or in books throughout your pregnancy, birth, and postpartum—or almost none of them. And that's okay.

One evening after a Birth Without Fear gathering, a mom approached me, tears quickly falling from her eyes as she introduced herself. She'd had a traumatic birth with her first baby, she told me. During labor, just as her body and her baby began to transition, she suffered a panic attack: out of control, disabling anxiety, heart pounding, struggling to breathe. "I'm pregnant with my second child," she said, "and I'm so afraid of that happening again." She explained that she had read everything she could get her hands on, but none of it addressed how to not have this happen again, and her fear would not subside.

"Will you have good support this time?" I asked her.

"Yes," she responded, describing her relationship with her midwife, doula, and partner. "But even with this team in place, nobody knows how to help keep me from experiencing another panic attack," she concluded.

"What if instead of trying to find something or someone that can keep your panic attack from happening again, you and your birth team *make space* for it to happen again?" I asked her. "What are some things you can tell your birth team to say or do that is comforting if it happens again? Make space for it to be *okay* for it to happen."

She had a look of shock on her face as this idea took root, and it was as if I could see this new perspective make sense to her in every cell of her body. She sighed, embraced me in a hug, and tearfully said, "Thank you. No one has suggested that but it makes so much sense."

We all have our own fears, our own stories like this woman's, our own histories we bring into pregnancy and birth. When I hear stories like this from parents all over the world, it always makes me wonder: Where did so many of us get this notion ingrained in us, that if we read or watch precisely the "right" combination of advice and information, if we plan and do everything "just right," that we can control the outcome or the journey to the outcome? Why do we put so much pressure on ourselves—pressure that can so easily turn to blame, self-hate, disappointment, and anxiety when the outcome isn't as expected?

You don't have to chase the elusive perfection. There is no "right" way. There is only your way, your baby's way, and your family's way. You can't control the pregnancy and birth journey—all you can do is make space for yourself. Get really interested in listening to and trusting your instincts. Don't fight yourself. Give yourself permission to feel whatever it is you're feeling each step of the way with love and acceptance.

The first trimester, which is usually considered to be the beginning 13 or 14 weeks of pregnancy, may include getting a positive test, interviewing care providers, having your first few appointments with your provider, and, perhaps, toward the end of this period, seeing or hearing the baby's heart tones for the first time. At this beginning stage, I encourage you to think of yourself as setting the foundation for a supported, affirming journey, so that you get the care, love, and support you deserve. And to do so, you need to know deep in your bones that you are worthy of respect, love, and care. Just as importantly, you need to be able to act from this belief when it comes to all those beginning things: choosing a care provider, announcing your pregnancy to family and friends, and navigating the changes in your body and moods. You deserve it not just for your baby but for *yourself*. The baby is important, and so are you.

Here's one of the weird and wild things about reproduction: during that interim period between ovulation and taking a pregnancy test, everything you're feeling could be a symptom of PMS *or* pregnancy. It can be infuriating or terrifying and really fray your nerves. Maybe even more so if you have a history of loss or infertility. You may get positive tests right away and you may not. Not everyone does. You may not feel anything until you've missed a period. If you've had additional pregnancies you may not even need a test: it's possible you'll feel an energy shift and just know something is different and have a pretty good idea what that something is.

Even after confirmation of pregnancy, there are plenty of variations of normal. You may have zero early signs—I hear a lot from women who think something is wrong when they don't feel anything in those first weeks, when you may just be less susceptible to feeling the hormonal changes. On the other hand, you may feel tenderness in your breasts and nausea right away. Both are variations of normal.

The first trimester is also the time when you may experience that much-dreaded—and much-misunderstood—symptom of pregnancy: morning sickness. For some, "morning sickness" would be a hilariously inadequate misnomer if you weren't feeling too sick to laugh. You may indeed feel nausea in the morning, but plenty of women experience it in the afternoon or the evening. You might feel sick all day, and not just in the first trimester but sometimes into the second trimester. And, I hate to say it, even throughout your pregnancy. I've been sick at every one of those points during some of my pregnancies. For some pregnancies, though, your normal may be little to no nausea at all.

During my first pregnancy, my first wave of morning sickness happened at Christmas *dinner*. My entire family was spending the holidays in the White Mountains of eastern Arizona. The nausea hit me during the thirty-mile drive from our cabin to the restaurant. Nothing sounded good at dinner, and the food I did eat did not want to stay down. Although my menstrual cycle was late, I was often irregular (and two previous pregnancy tests were negative), so I figured I just had a stomach virus. Nausea came over me every day for the next couple of weeks, sometimes in the morning, sometimes in the afternoon or at night. It took a while to figure out I was pregnant, as even a third test came back negative. I finally had to go to an OB/GYN to figure out what the heck was going on with me. At 9 weeks, I learned I was pregnant.

At no point during that first pregnancy did I get a break of more than a few hours from "morning sickness." I lost a total of thirty-five pounds. The midwives were worried I was losing too much weight, but that didn't concern me at all. I had some to spare.

I was not diagnosed with hyperemesis gravidarum (HG) during that pregnancy, but knowing what I know now, all the signs were there. HG is one of those things in pregnancy that is rarely talked about, and therefore it can be difficult to be taken seriously when you have it or think you do. It is characterized by extreme nausea and vomiting that causes weight loss and dehydration. Vomiting multiple times a day and feeling dizzy are the usual signs and symptoms. When looking into HG, most websites and doctors will tell you that it is extreme morning sickness that lasts up to twenty weeks before clearing up, and in some cases it may last longer.

Anywhere from 0.5 to 10.8 percent of pregnant women experience HG—it is not yet well diagnosed.[1] If you're working, making numerous trips to the bathroom to vomit, or taking sick days—days that you may be trying to save to use after your baby is born—it is very stressful. In addition to being told by your doctor or midwife to eat ginger and saltines and drink water, you may also be told to go outside for a walk or that it's just a case of mind over matter. It can be maddening to get a stock answer from your care provider, a person you are putting a lot of trust in to care for you during your pregnancy. It can feel like a condescending slap in the face. It's easy for depression to seep in and to feel like your entire world is spiraling out of control. I've been there.

At one point during my first pregnancy I was so sick and dehydrated that I found myself making several visits to the hospital for outpatient treatment to get intravenous fluids. During my fourth or fifth visit, I thought I might finally feel well enough to try a little food. The only thing I wanted was clear carbonated soda and a bite of a hamburger to see if I could keep them down. I took three sips and a bite or two of the burger that Brandon had brought, and that's all I could do. When the nurse came back in and saw the burger wrapper, she quickly turned judgmental, lecturing me about eating chicken and vegetables, or crackers and plain ginger. Obviously, this nurse knew very little about me, or she'd have known that the very sight of chicken even when I'm *not* pregnant makes me gag.

When you're really sick and trying to keep something—anything—down, a judgmental or inconsiderate response from a care provider can make you feel insecure. Instead of offering compassion and personalized care, they invalidate what you're going through. So often women's symptoms aren't taken seriously, and they are judged for what they do eat when they can. This is why finding a care provider who is competent and respectful is important—so that *you* are supported through your unique pregnancy (and birth). And if they are not knowledgeable or supportive, it's your right to change providers to one who is.

If you're not sick, however, it doesn't necessarily mean there's something wrong. There are no rules that say you have to have morning sickness or that morning sickness will only happen in the morning or only for *x* number of weeks. And there are exactly as many variations of normal for when you'll start showing as there are variations of bodies. If you're pregnant with your second or third (or fourth or fifth) child, know that your uterus is a badass muscle with a very good memory, so it's common to hear women say they start showing sooner with subsequent pregnancies.

There are many "normal" ways to *feel* when you become pregnant, too. Whether you've been trying to conceive for a while, you got pregnant immediately, or it was a complete surprise, pregnancy brings with it a whole range of emotions. It's easy to get caught up in trying to feel how you think you're *supposed* to feel instead of allowing yourself the freedom to acknowledge your feelings in all their complex (and even conflicting) messiness: excitement, fear, uncertainty, the desire to plan, the need to share your news, the longing to keep it all to yourself, residual feelings from previous pregnancies or life experiences. Sometimes I feel all those things just trying to remember to renew our vehicle registration and put the hummus away at night. So it's only natural that along with any physical signs, a flood of emotions will accompany pregnancy, one of those life-reorienting, existential human experiences.

Rather than trying to feel the "right" way about it, choose to let yourself fully experience it. Be on your journey. Let yourself ride a roller coaster of feelings and accept that things will change for you and your family. It's okay to be scared and excited and exhausted all at once.

Empowered Decision Making: Choosing a Care Provider

Your provider is a big part of your pregnancy. Regardless of who else you have on your birth team—a supportive partner, a fabulous doula, and so on—the truth is that your provider, whether they be an OB or a midwife, is a major partner in your birth journey. It's important that your relationship with your provider is one of trust and respect.

You are so awesome; make sure you have a care provider who knows how amazing you are. You are allowed to have a voice in your relationship with your care provider. You are at the start of a very long journey of advocating for yourself and for your children. You can start it at any time (and restart it at any time), and interviewing providers is one powerful way to do so.

In picking a provider, you don't have to go with your mom's gynecologist or limit your search to whoever is close by and is covered by your insurance. You're not going to know what's going to happen in every situation, so let go of that need to ask all the "right" questions or make the "perfect" pick right away. Instead, prioritize finding someone whose philosophy is in line with yours, whatever your situation. By interviewing providers, you're educating yourself and you're opening up a conversation to see if the two of you are a good fit together. Who's the person behind the credentials? Your goal is a working relationship based on respect and mutually aligned goals.

During your first and every appointment with your provider, you have the right to as much information as you need to feel at ease. And you have the right to a second opinion if you feel unheard, unseen, or disrespected—whether it's your first or tenth appointment. Even if something just felt "off." If your OB or midwife wants to do a cervical exam and that makes you uncomfortable, you are allowed to voice your discomfort and ask to discuss the practice of cervical exams with them. If your care provider is not taking seriously how sick you're feeling, you need to see someone else. If your care provider is part of a huge group of providers you'll never meet until one of them is on call when you go into labor, it's okay to get some assurances that you'll know the person who's there when you birth your baby. Trust your instincts from the beginning, because the more you shut off that voice the harder it gets to listen to it as you move along. You've got this one body, *your* body. The fact that you want to understand what's going on with it is not embarrassing or annoying. You have every reason to want to know yourself, to trust yourself and your provider, and to ask as many questions as you want about your body.

We have a misguided assumption as a society that providers "let" us do things. As a plus-size woman who has had VBACs and consistently goes 42-plus weeks, I was often—and by often I mean literally all the time—asked if my provider was "letting" me do that. This always confused me. I feel I have ownership of my body, not anyone else, and I was hiring a provider to *support* me, not control me. This is why it's important to know we have options and also to hire providers who will support us in our choices and respect us through the journey of pregnancy and birth. It's okay to voice concerns. If a provider has a policy you don't understand or agree with, ask them why—is it a hospital rule, or do they have a valid concern based on their experiences? When they want to introduce an intervention, you can ask for evidenced-based care.

Approach care providers with an open mind. Communicate in such a way that you make sure you are heard, but don't forget to listen, too. Your goal is an open discussion. If that isn't happening from the beginning, then that person is not the midwife or OB for you. Remember, your pregnancy and birth are and will be unique. Your purpose in interviewing care providers is to create a strong relationship. You don't want to fight with them over the weeks to come. Having a provider you trust and one who supports you will remove doubt when they have a concern or want to introduce an intervention, because sometimes interventions or changes to the plan are needed. What you want to eliminate by hiring the right provider for you are any insecurities and worries that they don't have a good reason for their suggestions and recommendations. You want a balance between evidence-based care and individual care, between their expertise and experience and your unique situation.

The following are some great questions to ask when interviewing providers:

- Are you planning to be in town around my due date?
- What is my certainty that you or your backup will be available for my labor?
- If your backup isn't available to attend my birth, what's the plan?
- Who else will be assisting you during my labor?
- What's your rate of cesareans?
- Do you practice regular episiotomies, and if I say no will you abide by my wishes?
- What laboring options do you support—tub, birthing ball, etc.?
- How late will you support me past my baby's estimated due date—both legally and personally?
- How many weeks are you comfortable with me going past 40 weeks? What is your reasoning behind your answer?
- How often do you do cervical exams, and will you support my choice to decline them if I decide at any time to do so?
- Do you support a family-centered cesarean—a cesarean birth planned in such a way that the birthing person feels part of the birth experience and immediately postpartum, with options for things like skin-to-skin contact following surgery and dropping the curtain or sheet so you can see your baby being born? Even if you are not planning one, it's good to ask to know what kind of provider they are and so you know your options if it does become a possibility or need.
- Do you have any questions for me?

If you're a VBAC birthing mama, you'll want to ask:

- Do you support a VBAC?
- What are your transfer rates from home to hospital?
- How many of your transfers have vaginal births and how many have cesareans? Why?
- If I go past 40 weeks, how long are you comfortable with?
- What are my options before a repeat cesarean?
- Do you support different labor positions other than lying on my back?

Other things you may start thinking about and discussing with your care provider (these will be discussed in greater detail when we talk about writing a birth plan):

- How do you and the hospital feel about delayed cord clamping?
- How do you and the hospital feel about skin-to-skin contact?
- What are your and the hospital's policies on delayed hepatitis B, vitamin K, and silver nitrate?

You can add many more questions to your list. We have an extensive list with comments on the Birth Without Fear website, and there are many resources available. The point is not to go into your appointment shooting questions like daggers at the care provider, but to calmly and respectfully open discussion to see if the two of you are a good fit. It's okay if you're not, and it's wonderful if you are.

If you live in a country where you don't get to interview providers, such as Canada or Australia, you can still fight for the care provider you know is best for you. You may need to look for loopholes, like going through a process where you self-refer to an OB or midwife if you don't have a good relationship with your family doctor and they aren't being respectful of that process. If you're finding yourself in a situation where you want a VBAC, you might have to fight for a referral to a VBAC-friendly OB or midwife. Although the medical systems are different, it's like the United States in the sense that sometimes you have to seek out alternatives if the care options you want aren't readily available to you. Don't be afraid to think outside the box.

Miscarriage and Infertility

This is not an easy topic—but I also feel that the more we treat it as taboo, the more alone we feel, when, in fact, infertility and miscarriage are common, shared experiences. As many as half of all pregnancies may end in miscarriage—in other words, it happens all the time.[2] They are variations of normal. That may not make your journey any easier, but you should know you're not alone. There's enough room to hold space for all circumstances, which includes loss, within the Birth Without Fear community. If, however, you're not in a space to read this, please skip to the next section.

Miscarriage is one of those experiences you cannot understand until you go through it. I did not understand the self-doubt or the feelings of shame that so often accompany miscarriage until I went through it myself. I had a miscarriage between my first two children that I chose to ignore. Call it a coping mechanism for my heart not being able to process or face it. I was not able to ignore my second miscarriage as easily.

One day, during a time when we lived in a small Texas panhandle town, we took the children into town to have a buffet lunch. After we had them all settled in with their favorite foods, I excused myself to go to the bathroom. When I wiped I noticed I was spotting. I thought it was my period, which was late, and thought no more about it.

A few days later my period still had not begun. I found it odd, but shrugged it off. The next day I thought I was finally beginning my period; however, after a few hours, something didn't feel right.

I was cramping more than usual and then my bleeding became very heavy. Soon I started passing large clots. I hadn't had a positive pregnancy test, so I didn't put it all together at first. I continued having this horrible period with cramping, clots, and serious exhaustion. I also felt off emotionally. That early evening it hit me. This was no period. I was having a very early "missed miscarriage." I felt deeply sad. My mind immediately went to self-doubt and blame. What did I do wrong? Am I getting too old? Did I do something I shouldn't have? Is my body just... broken?

I told Brandon and all he could do was express how sorry he was and that it would be okay. There wasn't much more he could do but be there for me emotionally.

My oldest daughter noticed I was sad and not feeling well. She asked me what was going on. She was ten at the time and I pondered whether or not to tell her the truth. I didn't want her to share the hurt I was experiencing, but at the same time she was also about to start puberty and I didn't want to pretend that this isn't common. It's a part of many girls' and women's lives. So I chose to explain to her what was happening. She quietly listened and thought about it. "So this would have been a baby?" "Yes," I told her.

The next day she asked if I could take her to the one and only coffee shop in town. Although I didn't feel up to it, I agreed. We sat there, me with my coffee and her with her salted caramel, as she asked me questions. I explained pregnancy and how sometimes this happens and there isn't always a reason. I tried to soften the sad feelings by explaining how it was so early on. She said, "So, this would have been my baby sister or brother." We both sat and silently cried together. After a few minutes she asked if she could look around the shop, which was also a boutique. She came back with this small, soft doll and asked if we could buy it to represent this baby we would not know. I was taken aback that she had thought of this on her own. Then she asked me something I was not expecting: "Can we name the baby?" Now, I wouldn't have personally done this on my own. Not with an early miscarriage.

But children don't make excuses to not process or feel how they do. I told her if she'd like to she could. She named our baby Dakota.

I've never shared this moment in any blog post or social media feed. It had a big impact on us, her holding space for this loss. You see, we had five children and we were "done." After processing this with my oldest daughter I had a discussion with Brandon. I told him she was right, this would have been another adorable Harshe baby. He agreed. Suddenly we were discussing whether or not we were really done. Brandon said, "Well, all children are a blessing and we make cute kids." I fell in love with him more in that moment. We decided to leave it open and you can guess how that ended. Our beautiful youngest child, our rainbow baby, was conceived seven months later. She makes us smile every day.

Struggles with infertility often also bring with them a self-worth issue, the feeling that your body is failing you or that your body is broken. I met a woman in Springfield, Missouri, who told me she had been trying to get pregnant for seven years. Dealing with infertility made it really hard for her to come to a place of body positivity, which was a prominent theme in the Birth Without Fear gathering she attended, "because," she shared, "I feel my body is betraying me." A few weeks later she messaged to tell me that she's finally pregnant, and then, sadly, she messaged me a week later to share that there was no heartbeat. On Mother's Day I wrote her to tell her I was thinking about her and sending her love and solidarity. I did so because we can and should support one another on our journeys even when they are different—not just the exciting parts, but the sad and difficult parts as well.

That day in the coffee shop, my daughter reminded me how important it is to allow yourself to feel how you feel, whatever that may be. It doesn't have to make "sense" to anyone, even to you. Give yourself grace to feel how you feel. It is okay to feel how you're feeling, to name your baby, to include her in the number of kids you have—and it is okay not to if that doesn't work for you. It's okay to be sad about one pregnancy and celebrate another. Whether the loss is late term or very early, you need to be validated in however you feel about the loss. If you've dealt with infertility before and are pregnant now, it's okay if this pregnancy, as ecstatic as it makes you, also makes your heart ache for all the times you tried to get pregnant before. Hold the space for yourself either way. If you feel alone in a loss or are struggling with overwhelming emotions, please reach out for support. I've included resources I trust at the end of this book.

Self-Care During the First Trimester

Self-care in the first trimester is about learning how to start choosing yourself and your baby first. How to advocate for you. It's more than a bath—although sometimes a bath is a damn good place to start—it's about taking care of yourself before others on your to-do list.

During the first trimester you may feel few to no changes and want to continue living your life exactly as usual, and that's great. It's also okay to start slowing down a little bit, or even a lot if you find you need it for any reason (if you have HG, for example, or if you crave the emotional and psychological support slowing down would afford you). You also don't need any reason at all, other than that is what you want to do. If your body is telling you to rest as it *literally creates a human*, take a nap or turn in early. If you are achy, take a bath or go for a swim. If you are feeling anxiety or more emotions than usual, make an extra appointment with your therapist or a date with your best friend for a coffee and vent session.

Give yourself the space to honor that you're creating a life. Just because you may not see or feel any overwhelming evidence of this fact doesn't mean that your body isn't still working overtime bringing cells together and making a person. If you don't believe me, go look up an embryology textbook. There's a lot going on!

You need to take care of you. Period. You don't need to justify or explain it to anyone (including yourself). Carve out a little extra space here and there on your calendar. Take five extra minutes to yourself in the morning before jumping on your phone or looking at your to-do list. Taking care of yourself is a practice or habit more than anything else, so start practicing how to fill your tank now. This practice will help you learn how to do so through this whole amazing journey you are on (for now, postpartum, and in parenthood). Laying a strong foundation for listening to your body and your instincts will serve you for your entire pregnancy, your birth experience, and postpartum—your whole life, really.

So often we feel we have to have permission to slow down and take care of ourselves. You don't need it. The thing is, you have every reason and right to listen to what your body needs already. I know that's easier said than done, so if you're the kind of person who tends to need permission from an outside source, I give you permission: while your body is making a tiny baby heart, you're allowed to take a nap or binge-watch Netflix. If the idea of "self-care" seems absolutely foreign to you and you don't know where to begin, I recommend starting with one small thing, like buying some pairs of underwear that fit, don't have holes, and aren't period panties.

It's also a good idea to spend some time thinking about when you want to announce. It's nice to wait and let these early weeks be a time for you, your partner, and your children, if you have them, to enjoy the beginning of things. Once you tell people you may quickly find that everyone—from family to random co-workers—will be in your business with opinions about your body and your pregnancy. Unsolicited advice (and even criticism) can come at you from all directions. Add to that the reality that we're the first generation to birth and parent in the age of social media, and the Pinterest-ification of pregnancy starts early with pregnancy announcements. Protect your space right from the start. Tell people you want to tell, but maybe save the Facebook status update for later so you can celebrate all over again with another circle of friends.

Start thinking about creating a bubble of support for yourself and your partner. Who's in, who's out? Take some time to take stock of the people in your life with clear-eyed honesty. One friend of mine is very close with her mother, but she also knows that her mother can be harsh, judgmental, and self-involved, and this triggers resentment and hurt in my friend. Acknowledging this doesn't mean she loves her mother any less or that her mother isn't an important member of her support team. It simply means she has the awareness to put boundaries on that relationship. When the conversation starts heading in a touchy direction, she knows to (politely) make her way to the door. She also knows she can address these issues head-on by saying out loud or to herself, "This is what I need from you right now. If you are unable to support me in this way I will limit our interaction." This is how your make your bubble—exploring how others make you feel and the kind of support and love the people in your life can give you through this journey, and putting yourself at the center of your own life.

It's hard enough to work through your own fears; it's hard enough growing a human. You don't need to deal with someone else's baggage, trauma, and fears. Who listens to you? Who empowers and supports you through decision making? Who makes it all about them? Who lectures and judges? Go all mama bear on it—anyone who doesn't support you gets a throat punch out of your bubble. Protect yourself just as fiercely as you would protect your baby.

PARTNER POINT OF VIEW:
Getting the News

January arrived home from work and handed me a small, neatly wrapped present for my twenty-fourth birthday. I had been on unemployment for a month and we didn't have much extra money at the time, so I was curious as to what was inside. I tore open the wrapping paper and stared at the gift for a moment, confused. It was a baby bath kit, complete with miniature bottles of baby shampoo, baby body wash, and baby bubble bath. *Why would I need this?* I thought. Then a worried notion entered my mind. Was our shampoo and body wash not working? Do I smell bad? I turned to January thoroughly confused, hoping she wasn't going to tell me I reeked. Instead, she simply said, "I'm pregnant."

I blinked.

Then, realization hit me. I stood up, my mind racing. I combed my fingers through my hair anxiously. *I'll need to get a job tomorrow,* I thought. *Definitely a second job by next week. Maybe even a third! Maybe I should rethink that chiropractic thing January mentioned a couple months earlier. I'd better enroll in classes for the next semester. We'll have to move out of this dinky apartment. How will I pay for the baby's college? How do I change diapers? How do I even hold a baby?*

"Are you happy?" she asked me hopefully.

I took a deep breath to calm my mind and assured January I *was* happy. I was simply trying to figure everything out, as if my life for the next couple decades would magically unfold before my eyes in that very moment. What I didn't understand then is that all the panicking I did in those first few moments, all the actions I thought I needed to take, and all the plans I wanted to make—they didn't matter. It wasn't about me. It was about our first baby. And considering our first baby was developing and growing inside of January, it was about her, too.

A positive pregnancy test is confirmation for your wife or partner that some of the feelings or symptoms she has experienced mean she is not losing her mind. She will experience more physical and emotional changes than she could ever imagine over the next nine to ten months as that baby grows and expands inside her womb. We partners will not, other than an occasional late-night trip to the grocery store for requested microwaveable taquitos and Ben and Jerry's.

The name of the game for partners is *support*. The pregnancy and eventual birth might not be real to you right now, but to your pregnant partner it is. Help her focus on the pregnancy and upcoming birth by focusing on her. And focusing on her means focusing on the pregnancy and upcoming birth *with* her.

Take a deep breath and enjoy the moment with your wife or partner. No need to plan out the rest of your life or your child's life just yet. There's plenty of time to do that, realize you had it all wrong, recalibrate, and repeat. Here is the reality: you'll learn, grow, and find your way into parenthood. There's no magic bullet, no job that will make everything perfect, no house that will solve all your problems, no one way of being or doing that will instantly make you a parent. It's a journey, and you get to go on it with the person you love most in the world, and you get to learn and unlearn and relearn how to do this together. Just allow yourself to grow on the journey of fatherhood.

Chapter 2

Advocating for Yourself:
Second Trimester Without Fear

....

*My beautiful friend, you deserve to be loved and supported
at your best, at your worst, and in between.*

You. Are. Powerful. You have a voice, intelligence, and an innate wisdom that is invaluable to your birth journey. You are not a statistic or a number on a scale, and you are not responsible for anyone else's baggage or fears. You, your baby, and your pregnancy are unique; you deserve unique, evidence-based care. You are your most valuable resource. You are the one who will be living, processing, and healing from your birth experience. The best advocate for you is you: listening to your intuition, working through your fears and anxieties, and surrounding yourself with people you trust.

I encourage you to think of the second trimester as a time for self-driven education: during these weeks you're going to be asked a lot of questions, faced with a lot of choices, and offered or encouraged to take a lot of tests. In order to be sure your voice is staying central to your journey, you are going to want to really educate yourself. There are so many resources available to help you do that. You may feel you have to read and listen to everything, which can be overwhelming, but remember that *you* get to choose what most empowers you in your decision making.

You may feel you'd rather go with the flow, free from expectations, unattached to any particular pregnancy and birth experience as long as you and your baby are healthy. Educating and advocating for yourself is a lot to take on while you're also growing a human! I understand that. I also agree with Melissa Bruijn and Debby Gould, authors of *How to Heal a Bad Birth*, however, that "the act of 'going with the flow' contains inherent pitfalls unbeknownst to most women who follow that plan of action. Unfortunately the question is not, 'Are you going to go with the flow?' In our current birthing climate, the real question is, 'Just whose flow are you going with?'"[3]

Going with the flow is a way of acknowledging the unpredictability of birth and a shared desired outcome for both you and your care provider: a healthy mom and baby. Yet too often "healthy mom and baby" does not prioritize your emotional and psychological health enough. Going with the flow will take care providers down whatever path leads to a healthy mom and baby, and that's great—but sometimes it comes at the cost of your voice and agency over your body. It should not be physical health prioritized over emotional and psychological health, or the other way around; all the above are important and should be considered. The things you do to strengthen your voice—educating yourself about testing, continuing to put together a supportive birth team, and prioritizing self-care—can help ensure that your voice is front and center throughout your journey.

I once spoke with a woman who had gotten an "intermediate risk" result on a test that may indicate things like Down syndrome and heart defects, called the nuchal test. Her midwife told her not to worry, downplaying her concerns; her doctor told her she absolutely had to undergo additional testing and should consider termination. She was terrified. Her friends only made it worse by moralizing about the blessing of having a child with Down syndrome and telling her not to worry. While this is certainly true for some families, her friends were missing the point, and so were her midwife and doctor: they were all telling her what to do instead of offering her information, discussing all the options, and supporting and respecting her decision making.

This is why it is so important that you advocate for yourself. As testing increases and your care providers begin playing a more prominent role in your birth journey, more variations of normal will surface. When something comes up as it did for this woman—you take a test with an unclear result or a test that requires another test—the most important thing is that you receive the information you need to make the best decision that's right for you without feeling shamed or judged.

The second trimester is usually considered to include weeks 13–14 through 27–29. During this time you may experience visible, tangible changes to your body, from swelling to heartburn to a growing "baby bump" and feeling your baby move for the first time. The second trimester is often the period in which testing is most prevalent. Many families will find out the sex of their baby during this time, too, while other families choose to stay "team green"—that is, not find out the sex until the baby is born.

Variations of normal during the second trimester may include what's called round ligament pain—a jabbing sensation in the lower belly or groin area as the ligament surrounding your womb tightens and stretches—and other sensations or discomfort as your baby grows. Uncomfortable, yes, but also normal parts of pregnancy growth. Or you may feel none of these. You may start showing during these weeks, or you may have started showing during the first trimester. Some women feel stretching on the sides of their bellies; others don't. You may feel exhausted—and you also may have bursts of energy and the desire for "nesting," which can mean everything from cleaning and organizing to refinishing furniture and painting rooms. If you have HG or morning sickness—and I know you may still be going through this and that the sickness didn't magically end at 12 weeks—I see you and I validate what you're going through.

Lots of women begin feeling their babies move between weeks 15 and 19, and variations of normal can range from as early as 13 weeks or not until into the 20th week. It's also possible that you won't feel much at all, and this can be due to the position of your placenta—if it is between you and your baby, which is referred to as an "anterior placenta," you're less likely to feel movement early or as often. Other things that can affect when you notice baby moving include being on the go with work or chasing a toddler around all day.

Many women feel physically and emotionally drained during the second trimester. A lot of physical and hormonal developments are taking place. You may feel a heightened sense of your emotions: noticing increased frustration, anger, sadness, excitement, and more. Maybe you feel overwhelmed or just *done* at work or with your toddler and partner. It's also a variation of normal if you don't feel especially emotional or uncomfortable at all. Your body, your emotional state, and your hormones are unique to you and this pregnancy. If you're dealing with physical and emotional strain—discomfort, nausea, anxiety, depression, and/or a needy four-year-old (and/or a ten-year-old, a pain in the ass boss, a nosy family member, etc.)—please take care of your physical and mental health. Say no to whatever you can say no to. Get a massage. See a chiropractor; chiropractic care can really help alleviate aches and pains. See your therapist or your best friend. Make an extra appointment with your provider to discuss only what is concerning you at this moment. Hide in the bathroom and read a magazine for twenty minutes. Go for a swim or a prenatal yoga class. And sleep. Always choose sleep.

If you don't love being pregnant, that's okay. I think sometimes we hear it said from our mothers or co-workers or whoever that the second trimester is the happy trimester—morning sickness is over but you haven't reached the uncomfortable big baby phase of late pregnancy. But that's just some people's experience. It's just a variation of normal.

Other variations of normal are perinatal depression, anxiety, or psychosis—they are real and they are debilitating, and you are not a failure if you experience them. You are not a failure if you feel sick, uncomfortable, or scared. Let go of whatever story you have about what pregnancy "should" be and give yourself permission to get the care you need. If none of these things—yoga, swimming, massage, sleep—are helping, and you don't feel that you can talk to anyone, that's a big clue that you *need* to talk to someone. Talk to a care provider if the depression, anxiety, or whatever else you're dealing with feels too heavy and isn't lifted with any of these suggestions or other things you try. No amount of prenatal yoga will magically balance your hormones if that's what you need. It's okay to ask for help. It's okay to say *I can't do this alone.*

With testing being so common during the second trimester, that means it's also a time when you're likely to have lots of questions and decisions to make. During my first pregnancy, I began feeling overwhelmed and more than a little frustrated with the number of tests that I was being offered. A good friend said to me, "It's not the tests that are the issue; you don't have to fight every test. It's what you're going to do with the information you're given." Six kids later, I know my friend was right: the problem with tests is usually not the tests themselves. It's the fear of what information they'll give us—or how a care provider may use that information to shame us or force a decision. One thing to keep in mind, though, is that it's not just *what* to do with the information you're given, but also *how* to deal with the stigmas and misconceptions that too often accompany testing and test results.

If you're a plus-size woman, you may be told you're at higher risk for all sorts of things, and if you're thin you may be assumed to be healthy and told that your physical concerns are all in your head. If you're a woman of color, you may have experienced having your pain or concerns downplayed, with no one ever acknowledging the effect shame and stress can have on the health of you and your baby. We have such amazing medical capabilities today, and yet it still needs to be said: care providers are human beings, who are educated and trained by a medical community with its fair share of limitations, especially when it comes to women's health. Sometimes stereotypes, myths, and assumptions drive the care we receive.

In light of this reality, how can you make sure you're receiving supportive, individualized care? Ask yourself this: Is my care provider giving me care with shame or without shame? A test and its results are important, but so is the feeling that your care provider respects you as an individual and a person. Are you receiving testing with shame or without shame? Are the results of testing being delivered to you with a judgmental tone, or is your care provider simply sharing information and your options, and supporting you?

When a care provider asks you to do a test, it is absolutely always okay for you to ask why. If they want you to test for something based on your weight, then a frank discussion needs to happen, or it's time to change providers. If your provider has set limitations on your VBAC plan, ask for evidence-based reasons. Why are they asking for it? Why are they setting limitations? Are they judging you? Or are they concerned? When the testing is being done, are you getting comments from the staff about your weight or your small pelvis? Testing should come from a place of making sure you and baby are healthy, and with the goal of preparing for the best outcome for you both—and not from a place of fear. Remember this: part of the "best outcome" includes you being treated with respect.

Testing for gestational diabetes, which is done during the second trimester, is one of those tests largely shrouded in misconceptions and stigma. Although gestational diabetes is caused by diet and not by how much you weigh, many women are judged by their care providers based on their size.[4] As a plus-size post-date VBAC mom, I was frequently told I'd have gestational diabetes. I didn't. Not once in all six of my full-term pregnancies. We hear story after story in the Birth Without Fear community of doctors and midwives assuming plus-size women will develop gestational diabetes and that their plans to labor in water or without medication are unreasonable unless they lose weight. And we hear just as many stories of thin women shocked that they have been diagnosed with gestational diabetes after being told they were not at risk due to their weight. This is not individualized or even evidence-based care; it is care given with judgment, assumption, and shame.

We need to break through the body shaming not only when it comes to gestational diabetes but also to weight and body size in general throughout pregnancy and birth. I've heard from many women who are told by their care providers after miscarriage that they'd have better luck next time if they lost weight. This is body shaming, not true, and not supportive care. I would have been "risked out" at birthing centers because of my BMI. There is a huge stigma regarding body size in our culture that becomes even more prevalent when a woman is pregnant. The stigmas are deeply rooted and unfortunately experienced through comments, looks, and the way care is given by care providers and their staff. If only many of them realized that they could make an incredibly powerful shift in the care they give! Until this shift happens, if we cannot find a provider who gets it, we must be our own best advocates for dispelling these myths by expecting and insisting on care without shame.

During my sixth pregnancy, I chose to do co-care with a midwife and an OB. On one visit to my OB, the nurse, whom I'd never met before, called me in and took me right to the scale. I politely said "no," and then gestured toward my body in Vanna White fashion and said, "See all this? I'm good with this." She appeared flustered and did her best to convince me I had to be weighed. But I stood my ground. "It has taken me a long time to love myself in my body and there is nothing that that number is going to determine about my care and my baby's care. *If* you need to give me an epidural I'll let you know how much I weigh. That's on a need-to-know basis."

She must have understood my determination because she nervously replied, "I'll just write 'patient refuses' on your chart."

"I'm not gonna be weighed for you. There is no reason you need an exact number of how much I weigh today," I told my OB a few moments later in the exam room, and he laughed, because he knew me and totally understood. Because you know what? My cervix and my vagina never asked me what my BMI was.

Many of us work really hard to feel good about ourselves and in an instant a careless comment, an assumption about our weight determining some outcome, or a number on a scale—and don't get me started on the nonsense that is the BMI—fills us with shame or doubt because of our size, whether we're being told our pelvis is too small or our body is too big. And that's how we're being judged, not for our whole selves or for the full spectrum of our health, but for our size. It can undermine the authority of your inner voice. To that I put both middle fingers up and wave them high. Your size is a variation of normal. Your weight doesn't determine your health; your health determines your health.

Empowered Decision Making: Preparing for Birth

The second trimester is a good time to start thinking about your birth experience: who to have with you on your birth team, including your care provider, whether or not to hire a birth doula and a postpartum doula, and where and how you want to birth. You had some appointments and conversations with care providers during your first trimester, and once you reach the second you'll want to start making those interviews more official. As you have your visits and your questions come up, you'll have plenty of opportunities to find out if your visions align, and by the end of the second trimester, ideally you'll have it worked out so that you won't make changes during the third trimester, although that happens—I've done it or been forced to do it more than once—and if it does, it doesn't mean you've failed; the system that we have to birth in sometimes fails us.

By the time you're ready to hear the baby's heartbeat and start thinking about what kind of birth experience you want, it's time to set up interviews and consultations with care providers. You're looking for someone who works *with* you. You want their insight.

You want their perspective. You'll ask for their opinion. You're looking to them for their expertise. They're not the boss of you. You're partners. You're building on your first trimester bubble of support. You're creating a birth team.

Here's what I mean when I say "birth team": you've got yourself, maybe a spouse or partner (or mom or best friend), and maybe even a doula—and then you bring in your care provider on that same level. So often we think of ourselves as either subordinate to medical experts, or, when we're trying to flip that script, we think of ourselves as the boss of our care providers—that they are subordinate to us. But all of this is so linear and businesslike. It's emblematic of our modern society to think this way. Birth isn't a business relationship, and it's not a hierarchy. It's a partnership, a team. It's a journey and a life transformation. Everyone needs to work together in an open and trusting way. You wouldn't want to put your doctor above you but you wouldn't want to put them below you either. Same goes with your partner. Just like the bubble of support I talked about in chapter 1, it's not a hierarchical relationship—it's a circle, a feedback loop in which each person weighs in, is heard, and discusses options together.

I recently heard from a woman who was experiencing pain in her abdomen. She saw her OB, who told her it was round ligament pain, but after her appointment she felt that little voice of instinct telling her the pain was something more, something different. "I had round ligament pain with my first pregnancy, and this didn't feel the same. I didn't want to bother them," she said, "but I called in anyway. My OB wasn't there and the person on call treated me like an idiot. I know they're busy." Unfortunately, it's so easy to silence those little voices of concern inside yourself if you feel unhappy with or unheard by your doctor. You have a legitimate concern about your body or your pregnancy, and yet you feel as if you're bugging your care provider when you call or go in for an appointment. This is not a supportive provider or partnership. If your midwife makes you feel scared about a test result and then ignores you when you share how their comments made you feel, this is not a supportive provider. On the other hand, if you find yourself constantly arguing with your care provider and questioning everything they say, that's not supportive care for you, either. These providers don't belong on your team. They don't belong in your bubble of support.

Make your birth team or bubble whatever it needs to be for you. If you are a single parent, your support person may be your best friend, parent, or doula. And then, maybe overlapping or just faintly touching that bubble, there is everyone else. Be intentional with where you place people. Maybe your parents, your sister, and your knitting group are in another bubble, close by but not on the team.

Sometimes women at events will ask me when we're going to get better national policies to support women and families from the highest levels of government. I don't think these changes happen from the top down (although that would be nice); we need to do this in our own communities. We don't have time to wait for the system to change, and it won't happen all at once; we have to make waves and changes however we can, and now. We need to be like those little old ladies gossiping about who's doing what and how. Building a birth team can be daunting, I know. But you don't have to start from scratch. If you find a birth doula you love, ask them for OB or midwife recommendations; if you find an OB or midwife you love, ask them for doula recommendations. Ask your closest ICAN (International Cesarean Awareness Network) group—even if you're a not a VBAC mama. They know who the good providers are. Ask your friends. Make your sources of information not just books and articles, but also other women's stories. There is something very powerful about sharing our experiences and building coalitions and networks of good providers from there.

You might be interested in inviting a doula into your bubble to help everyone on the team get through it. Doulas are amazing because they get to know you, your partner, and your family through your pregnancy. They offer support and a wealth of knowledge. Women will often say that they want their partner to support them in labor, or that they don't want to share their birth experience with a stranger. But who supports the partner? Who is an advocate for them both when shifts change in a hospital birth or when plan A isn't quite working? This is where having a doula can be a great comfort: they're there to be a support for everyone no matter where your journey takes you.

Doulas technically can't advocate on your behalf to your OB or midwife, but your partner absolutely can, and a doula can help a partner use their voice. In addition to helping partners help laboring mamas, doulas can help laboring women remember all the things they wanted for their birth experience. Think of a doula as an outside person with experience and knowledge who will be with you all the time to help you remember all the things you wanted and to give you emotional support throughout your pregnancy and postpartum; physical support in the form of hip squeezes, massage, suggesting position changes, and heat and ice packs; and information to help you make decisions for yourself.

Some women know they want a particular doula, and, in order to make sure they get who they want, will hire that a doula as early as 8 weeks—or some before they're even pregnant! But unless you have that level of clarity and specificity, the second trimester is a great time to start interviewing doulas. Just as with anyone on your birth team, you need to interview doulas to determine whether hiring a doula is right for you and, if so, find one with whom you connect. During interviews you can learn more about what doulas offer in general and the unique philosophy and personality of each doula you talk to. A doula is there to support *you* and your partner or spouse, so finding someone who fits well on your team is important. And just as with care providers, if at any point that relationship becomes a burden or stress on your birth journey, it's okay to fire your doula. It's also okay not to want one.

The second trimester is also a good time to start thinking about where and how you want to birth: a home birth or a scheduled cesarean, a hospital birth, or in the woods by a baby deer (yes, I've actually seen this in a birth photo of a mom laboring outside with her partner in a Jacuzzi tub). Are you interested in a water birth or laboring in the water? Are you interested in squatting to birth your baby out? We'll include lots more information on choosing an OB/GYN in the chapter on hospital births, on midwives in the home birth chapter, and on supportive providers for women hoping to have a vaginal delivery after cesarean in chapter 6. But, for now, it's a good idea to start thinking about where and how you'd like to birth, and doing some self-education.

If you're interested in midwives and you find a local home birth midwife, you may want to schedule an interview in your home. If you find a birthing center midwife, you'll probably do an interview in the birthing center and take a tour of the facility. If you want to birth with a hospital-based Certified Nurse-Midwife (CNM—a registered nurse who has completed an accredited graduate-level nurse-midwife program and is certified by the American Midwifery Certification Board) or OB practice, check to see if they host a monthly meet and greet you can attend, or call and ask to schedule a consultation to meet and see if the provider aligns with the type of birth you're envisioning. In this case, specify that you're scheduling a consultation and not going in for a checkup (some practices will charge for these; some won't). It's nice to keep those separate. Don't be afraid to ask for a consult. A doctor does not need to put their hand in your vagina or weigh you just for you to ask them some questions about your care.

If you know you're hoping for a VBAC, you'll want to specifically ask if that provider is supportive of VBACs, and in the event of a cesarean birth, it's helpful to ask if they are supportive of family-centered cesareans. Depending on your unique situation, you may also want to ask any care providers you interview if they are size-friendly, LGBTQIA-friendly, and anything else that's specific to you: previous traumas, for example, or health issues or concerns.

I mentioned earlier that with my sixth pregnancy I chose to do co-care with a midwife and an OB. Since I sometimes wish someone had told me I could make such creative and self-supportive decisions with my earlier pregnancies, I'm here to tell you: you have options. You can ask for just about anything you think will work for you—maybe it's not possible, but it doesn't hurt to explore. I often hear from women who are under the care of midwives that if they have to transfer to an OB or a hospital, they feel abandoned by their midwives. The benefit of arranging co-care is that you develop relationships with a range of care providers. When I had my cesarean birth with co-care, my midwives visited me in the hospital and did my postpartum follow-up at home. When I thanked my midwife for continuing to care for me, she seemed confused. "I transferred care to my OB when I chose a cesarean," I explained. My midwife responded, "Well, you're still our client. And it seems to me that if you transfer you might need us more with recovering, healing, processing, and breastfeeding." This is the kind of full-spectrum care and support we all deserve.

Keep co-care in mind when you're interviewing care providers. The choices available to you for co-care will likely depend on where you live and the laws of your state, as well as each individual practice. But you can always be creative! Some practices have co-care built in: a group that includes both midwives and OBs, for example. Some birthing centers have to be overseen by OBs, depending on state regulations. For me, I found a midwife I liked and, since they didn't have OBs they worked with or referred to, I found an OB I liked—and I made sure that they were each okay with the fact that I was seeing the other. You'll also have to explore payment options with co-care: Can you afford both care providers? Is either or both willing to help you figure out a payment plan that works for you? Can they help you find out if your insurance works in this situation? It may take some extra planning and imaginative thinking, but if it helps you feel empowered and supported, it's worth it. You are worth it.

Self-Care During the Second Trimester

The second trimester is a bridge—a magical unicorn bridge—between the first and the third. As you near your baby's birth day in the third trimester, you'll be focusing your energy on creating and maintaining your space like a fierce mama bear. The more you educate yourself, acknowledge and address your own fears, and listen to your intuition during the first and second trimesters, the more confident you'll be not allowing other people's fears into your birth when the time comes.

Here's what I do with my own fears: I ask myself, Is this something that I'm afraid of because of a birth story I read or something that happened to a friend or to me in a previous experience—or is it my instincts telling me that I should look into it more? In other words, is the thought in my head a fear or an instinct—a voice of anxiety or intuition? Anxiety is a liar, but intuition is precisely the voice you want to strengthen and empower.

Anxiety can often be eased with more and better information. If you are scared of something, that just means it's something you need to learn more about. You can always educate yourself more and ask more questions. If it's your instincts that are nudging you, do what you need to do: get a test, talk to your provider, or get a second opinion. And if you just aren't sure, it's okay to always get whatever is bothering you checked on. Remember your bubble of support and the circle of your birth team—this is *your* team, your support network, and at any point you should be able to turn to them to help alleviate your fears and anxieties. If you're going through anxiety and you have fears, that's what your birth team is there for.

You can also use your instincts to guide you when it comes to revealing your baby's gender, your due date, and even how far along you are. Keep in mind the importance of creating your space: sometimes you want to share everything and sometimes you want to keep things to yourself. Only you can decide how much to reveal and who you want to let in.

Once people know your baby's gender, a whole lot of input tends to follow. I remember one woman bemoaning how often people told her "a girl steals your beauty" after her gender reveal. I'd never heard that one before and it confused me...why is there not enough beauty to go around? How exactly is that supposed to be helpful? It's the same for due dates—inevitably someone will comment on how "big" you are or aren't, give opinions on how you should or shouldn't birth, and offer other unnecessary commentary. I used to tell people who asked how far along I was: "somewhere between 20 and 60 weeks."

When you start showing, you may also find that people start touching your belly. By "people" I mean anyone from close friends and family to strangers at the bus stop or in line at the store. It can be very strange to suddenly feel you've lost your personal boundaries. You may not mind people touching your belly, or you may feel it's a violation of your space and body. Both are variations of normal. In a perfect world, a person would always ask before touching your body, but since we don't live in a perfect world, take care of yourself when it comes to maintaining your space.

We tend to feel we owe people—even people we don't know—the truth about the intimate details of our bodies and lives. Or that pregnancy somehow gives others unfettered access to our bodies. I'm here to tell you: you don't owe anyone anything. Tell people as much or as little as you want to tell them. Say "no, thanks" or protect your belly with your arm when someone touches you—or put your hand on their belly until they realize how weird they're being! This is your space, your body, your journey.

I've been talking a lot about the circular nature of your birth team and your bubble of support, and despite the importance of creating that safety net around you, it's also normal if you have moments of feeling alone in your journey. The changes are happening to *your* body, after all, and at the end of the day, once family and friends go home and your partner is asleep, it can feel as if you're the only one really present to this new life growing. I've been there; I understand that feeling. I'm here to encourage you to ask for the help you need. This is the heart of good self-care.

Sometimes you need to just sit with it and be in the moment. Take a deep breath and acknowledge that you are in the midst of a time of growth and change, and it's okay to feel whatever you're feeling. Everything doesn't have to feel great all the time. It's okay if you're not okay sometimes. You're not "supposed" to feel any certain way—you just feel how you do and that's a variation of normal. Reach out to the people in your bubble or bring in another support person if needed. None of us wants to be a burden to others, but sometimes we're just too damn good at pretending everything is fine. Better to tell a trusted friend what you're going through than to resent them later because they didn't know or understand. You deserve to be heard and held. You deserve to give yourself (and to have your team give you) the space for whatever comes up. Your feelings are valid and your mental health is worth it.

PARTNER POINT OF VIEW:
To Support and Be Supported

As the partner of a pregnant woman, it can be easy to lose sight of the struggle she goes through on a seemingly minute-by-minute basis. You aren't the one experiencing hormonal changes. You don't experience the discomfort of shifting organs because of a growing uterus. You won't experience the sharp pains in your pubic bone or round ligament areas. You probably aren't getting short of breath just walking from your bedroom to the kitchen. You're probably sleeping fairly well because you don't need to get up seven times during the night to pee. Comparatively speaking, you have it pretty easy in the physical department.

Sure, stepping up and taking on more responsibilities—making dinner, doing the dishes, getting kids bathed and ready for bed, doing the grocery shopping, rubbing her feet, and running her a bath are all fantastic ways to show your support for her. But there is so much more to pregnancy than just the structural and biological changes taking place. Emotionally, your partner might feel very alone. Yes, millions of other women are pregnant throughout the world at the same time as your partner, but that doesn't change the fact that she is the one going through this pregnancy, at this time, with your child. She will need you to comfort her and let her know everything will be alright, that she is doing great, and that you believe in her and the choices she's made for her pregnancy and birth experience. Even if you aren't completely on board with her choices, she deserves your support as her partner and future co-parent of that baby. It doesn't matter if she appears confident in her choices at all times. She is human, and humans have a tendency to experience some level of self-doubt now and then. Knowing that you are by her side supporting her 100 percent will only add to her confidence that the struggles of pregnancy are worth it and that she can do this, that she will do this.

One aspect of the pregnancy and eventual birth experience that partners don't often think about is who will be there to support *you*? There is a lot of work involved to make sure your significant other is taken care of and supported emotionally and physically. But what about you? If you're anything like me, the thought of another baby isn't tangible during the pregnancy. Yes, you know the baby is coming, but the baby is not here yet and you're the kind of person who goes by the old adage of "seeing is believing." Suddenly, your partner is moaning through contractions, then screaming and breathing heavily, that baby's head is crowning, and you're wide-eyed and panicked and unsure of what to do.

She will need your support during the birth, just as she does during pregnancy. No one will have her best interests in mind more than you, the partner. Not the doctor, not the nurses, not the anesthesiologist, not the midwife, not the assistant midwife. No one is invested in her health and well-being the way you are, because no one loves her the way you do. She may need you to be her advocate during the birth and to speak up if there is deviation from the birth plan. She will only get this one birth experience with this baby (or babies), but in the heat of the moment when she's exhausted or in pain and wanting the birth to simply be over, your job is to be there and let her know she can do it and that you believe in her, just as you've been doing all pregnancy long.

This is where a doula can take some of the load off your shoulders so that you can fully concentrate on being the teammate your partner needs during labor, transition, birth, and postpartum. A doula can't advocate for your partner the way you can, but a doula can certainly assist you in advocating. Being by your partner's side as she gives birth to your baby while doctors and nurses or midwives attend to her can be a bewildering, deer-in-the-headlights moment for you. A doula can help you avoid feeling this way by letting you know what your partner needs from you in those moments. Sometimes an outsider's perspective can be the balance needed to offset your emotional investment in the situation.

Start interviewing doulas with your partner now. Birth is a once-in-a-lifetime experience; no two births are the same, no matter how many kids you have. You want to find a doula you mesh well with, and one you know you can count on to be levelheaded and helpful when the big day arrives.

Chapter 3

Your Body Is Amazing, Your Baby Is Wise: Third Trimester Without Fear

· ·

At the end of pregnancy, it feels like time slows down to almost a screeching halt. You're now experiencing the beginning of your baby's birth story in real time. Sit with it. Be in the moment.

Breathe. Simply breathe. Take a deep breath in and slowly let it go. You have made it to the third trimester of your pregnancy. Your body is strong and capable. Your baby is wise. Breathe. You are in a time of growth and transition. Just be there. Be in your own strength. Tune into your inner voice, that deeper essence of you. What are your body and baby telling you? What are you supposed to learn through this? Only you can find that answer.

Now pause. Take a step back, even if for just a few precious moments. The reason every day probably feels like a year is because you're waiting for your birth experience and your baby's birth story to begin—but the truth is, you're already in it. You're in the beginning of your baby's birth story. We as a culture seem to believe birth starts when contractions begin or water breaks, but this notion only takes certain visible measurable markers as signs of birth. It ignores that hormonal, physical, and emotional changes are happening all along, and it ignores the innate intelligence of both you and your baby. But you don't have to ignore that intelligence—you can choose to honor it.

During the third trimester, changes can seem to increase exponentially. You may not notice any changes at the start of the third trimester, and then you may wake up one day around week 32 and think, "Oh, crap, in about five weeks I'm gonna be considered full-term. This is really happening." Checkups move from once a month to every two weeks, and around 36 weeks you're going every week. By the end of the third trimester, everything seems to speed up and slow down all at once. There can be so much restlessness during this time. Restless sleep, impatient and excited waiting, wondering who your baby will look like and what the birth will be like, and for some reason everyone everywhere keeps asking, "Have you had that baby yet?"

You can't rush time and you can't slow it down. Give yourself and your body the space to prepare for *your* birth experience while also giving your baby the space to have *their* birth story. Stop waiting for your water to break and give yourself permission to create a protective cocoon around you *now*; take some deep breaths and acknowledge that this is a time of transition, honoring the journey and whatever emotions it may bring. Don't think just about processing your own fears but also about not allowing other people's fears into your own space.

After my third birth, a hospital VBA2C (vaginal birth after two cesareans), I took a lot of time processing my three births and what led to the outcomes of those births. Not just how baby entered the world from my body, but each labor, the decisions that were made, how I was treated, and how postpartum went. I came to one very clear realization: that it wasn't just my fears (or trust) that affected my labors and births, but also the fears of my providers and the birth team present. It felt as if I couldn't find a care provider who had faith in me and my body. I spent all forty-plus hours of labor worrying about *their* fears and what they thought. I just wanted to birth a baby. I kept coming back to the knowledge of all the women before me who had birthed their babies. I felt a kinship with them.

I knew I could do that too. I no longer felt okay with care providers telling me I couldn't because I was plus-size, had had previous cesareans, or gone postdates. I was done with others doubting my ability when I wasn't doubting myself one single bit. I knew I could do this. I knew I could squat and push a baby out of my vagina without all the doubts, fears, and trauma.

For me, at the time of my fourth pregnancy, the only way I felt I could have this cocoon of support and trust was with an unassisted birth. It was one of the most empowering moments of my life. It was also a deeply healing experience, not just for me but also my husband. He says it was the best day of his life catching his baby girl with us surrounded by strength, trust, and love. But I don't want you to feel the way I did, that the only way you can birth is if you're backed into a corner, surrounded by everyone's opinions and yet at the same time feeling completely alone. I don't want you to feel that the only way to have a trauma-free birth is to do it alone. I don't want anyone doubting your ability to know and trust your body, especially when you aren't doubting your ability. Unassisted birth is an option and our right over our bodies and experiences, but it should not feel like your only option to have a supported, trauma-free birth. Women deserve options, respect, and support.

What I learned from my fourth birth is that no matter how you choose to birth, you must unapologetically protect your birth space, and that starts in the third trimester. Other people's energy and voices can so easily get into your head. Not allowing other people's fears and baggage into your birth space may come naturally to some people, but for others it takes practice. The more you educate yourself, speak up for yourself, and demand respectful and supportive care, the more you feel the effects of that and the more you will want it. It may be as simple as answering, "It's not up for discussion." with nosy family. It may be as much as switching to a doula who is a better fit for your birth space. It may be just needing space to feel however you feel and letting that be okay.

The third trimester is usually from around weeks 27–29 through weeks 40–42, with variations of normal going as much as 44 weeks. In fact, even the American Congress of Obstetricians and Gynecologists says that women are not to be considered postdates until they've reached the full 42 weeks.[5]

Variations of normal may include endless discomfort in your hips, joints, and muscles, or being too uncomfortable to get much sleep and getting up to pee all through the night. I can say from experience that the feeling of your baby kicking and moving inside you never gets old, no matter how many kids you have; and I can also say with confidence that many of us hit 36 weeks and we're done. Just. Done. Done with being pregnant, done with preparing for the baby, done with decision making, done! You may want your body back—not in the "pre-baby" body sense because that's not how I roll, but in the sense that you want to have your body physically back to yourself.

Remember: your body is amazing, your baby is wise, and you are at the beginning of your baby's birth story. Once your baby is in your arms, time will speed up so fast you'll barely be able to keep up. Try to enjoy this slowed-down phase for what it is, as you only have a little longer of it being just the two of you. And if just reading "try to enjoy it" makes you want to throw this book across the room, then I'll tell you this: just make space to feel however you f*cking feel because it's okay to do so.

Writing a Birth Plan Philosophy

By the third trimester of pregnancy, many women are ready to be done with all the logistical work: you've read all the research and maybe even prepared the nursery or co-sleeping space. Now you're just trying to get a few hours of sleep before the baby comes. I get that. Yet the third trimester is a great time to write what I call a birth plan philosophy. I know it's become common practice to write birth plans, but I think the word "plan" alone can be damaging—it can set up false expectations that you can plan for birth. It's good to plan, but things may not go as planned. A philosophy is how you feel about your intended birth experience. I would encourage you to create something that uses a little bit of both! Your plan focuses on certain logistics—delayed cord clamping, for example—and your philosophy lays out how you expect to be treated and the vibe you'd like to create for your experience. Think of writing this plan/philosophy as a way to get more comfortable knowing your options and solidifying your bubble, and a practice of keeping others' fears out of it while exploring your needs during labor and birth.

Writing a birth plan philosophy is both practical and imaginative. It is making your birth philosophy clear to you and your birth team. It allows you to make space for your emotional health during birth. A birth plan isn't a set-in-stone plan, because you can't possibly predict or control everything about birth. Rather, it is a tool for education, options, and support. It's about educating yourself further, looking into your options, and discussing them with your care provider to see if you're on the same wavelength. You'll want to let go and be in the flow during your birth, and writing a birth plan helps you feel confident that everyone on your team knows your preferences and is listening to your voice while you're busy laboring.

A written birth plan philosophy is a tangible expression of the kind of care you want and need. It clarifies for you and your team the kind of experience you want to have, no matter the specifics of your labor—unassisted, cesarean, hospital, home birth, birthing center, or even in the case of a transfer from one to the other. How will you find comfort? How can those present help support your confidence? What are your medication preferences? Your movement preferences? Your infant-feeding preferences? Your desires for skin-to-skin contact and cord clamping? Your feelings about episiotomy and placenta delivery?

It's crucial to take into account your emotional and psychological health when writing a birth plan. How can you create a safe and supportive bubble for yourself during labor and birth? How would you ideally like decisions to be made? What would improve your emotional health in the event that you need a cesarean birth? Or if a healing birth *is* a planned cesarean, is your birth team on board with your desires for a family-centered or maternal-assisted cesarean?

So many women and families tell me they are not writing a birth plan because they want to "go with the flow"—and then they add, "I wanted to try laboring in water" or "I was always interested in an unmedicated birth." But how will anyone know what you want and are interested in if you don't specify your preferences? This opens you up for the very real possibility that your voice will get lost in labor. Birth plans are wonderful not only for educating yourself (and your partner) but also to discuss with your provider to make sure you are on the same page. It's crucially important for your birth team to support your needs to help avoid birth trauma.

Writing a birth plan and philosophy is also a great conversation starter with your care provider. Go over it with them and ask questions. When a friend who had a traumatic birth with her first baby began talking to a new care provider about her birth plan for her second, he suggested picking a date to induce her as a way to ease her anxiety about the loss of control she experienced previously. She didn't like the idea of induction, and he respected that. But this conversation gave her an appreciation of her care provider's creative thinking and willingness to support her emotional health and to give her individualized (or unique) care. It showed her that they were a team, that they could have an open discussion not just about healthy baby and healthy mom, but also how to make sure she felt seen and heard. Writing a birth plan or philosophy helps open up these conversations and makes space for your voice.

Care Providers

It surprises a lot of women then that when they hit 30 and 40 weeks plenty of new things start coming up with their care providers;

sometimes brand-new things, sometimes things previously discussed and agreed upon by you *and* your care providers. If you've decided on a hospital birth, for example, it can feel like you're suddenly getting blindsided with policies and restrictions that hadn't come up before. Or if you've been planning to birth at home or in a birthing center, you may hear for the first time about restrictions based on state laws or practices once you reach 39 weeks. Many women become frustrated and overwhelmed with decisions they feel underprepared for during the third trimester, stuck wondering after weeks of planning and preparing, is everything changing?

What I hear all the time from women in their third trimester is that they come out of appointments with their care providers with more questions than they went in with. A doctor or midwife will say something off the cuff and unexpected, suggesting a new test or referring to a hospital policy not mentioned before, and so often women get home and find themselves fixated on it. "I'm thirty-nine weeks, I'm tired, and I'm frustrated. Should I get the membrane sweep?" "And also, what is a membrane sweep?" (Hopefully you don't have a provider who pressured you into a cervical exam or did one without even asking. Yes, it happens.) "I'm getting close to postdates; what does that mean?" "My doctor wants to do a nonstress test; what is it and should I agree to it?" "Should I try to get things moving, or should I slow things down?" When your focus should be on resting and protecting your space, this can become a distraction leading to frustration and anxiety. In your third trimester, your baby and your exhaustion are both growing. It's a good time to remember what *you* want and to make the space for your needs in the midst of what can feel like the ground shifting out from under you.

Lots of women are hesitant to call their care providers with what they're afraid are silly questions, and often for good reason: a call to your care provider usually means being put through to the nurse on call and then being told the doctor will give you a call back. When you do get called back, more often than not you're given a generalized answer or you get the feeling you're bothering them for asking.

Yet my first response to these kinds of questions is always: call your provider. Why? Because you deserve as much information as you desire and because it's your right to ask as many questions as you have. And because, believe it or not, the third trimester is often the time when red flags start to appear with your care provider, OBs and midwives alike, so it's also a great time to put that relationship to the test. If you're not getting helpful answers or if you don't feel heard, that's worth paying attention to. *You* have autonomy over your experience and you don't owe anyone your continued support or patronage if you don't feel completely at ease.

When talking to your care provider, it's a good idea to try to meet them where they are. Sometimes we need to stand our ground and blaze a trail to change policies and the care women receive, but always balance that instinct with protecting your space; you don't need to create more of a struggle for yourself. Understand that hospitals and birthing centers have standard operating procedures and that they tend to want everything running smoothly according to a particular standard of normal. The person on the phone with you may not have much power or may have never been asked questions like the ones you're asking. There may be certain instances where your provider will be comfortable in deviating from their standard protocol and certain instances where they will not. Maybe you don't want repeated cervical checks and ultrasounds near the end of a pregnancy, but you also know that your midwife or OB won't discontinue care with you if you pass your 42nd week of pregnancy as nearly every other care provider you interviewed would. An ultrasound during week 41 and/or 42 to alleviate any concerns your provider has might be a necessary compromise.

"Here's what I heard you say," you might ask your care provider. "What does that mean?" "What are my options?" "What's the hospital policy and why is it policy?" You can also ask to see the policy: "Can you show it to me in writing?" I've found that very often stated policies are not written anywhere, it's just how something has been done and the person you're talking with isn't willing or able to go against the status quo. If it's not a written policy, you are well within your rights to keep pushing for what you want. I've had wonderful nurses tell me they love it when their mamas do this.

If the policy in question is in writing, you get to decide if you are going to push back anyway. Do you feel there is a good reason for this policy? Is it something you are willing to compromise on? Do you want to push back? Or is this policy a reason to find a different care provider, a different hospital, or a different birthing center?

Meeting your care provider in the middle does not mean compromising on all things, and especially not when they reverse course on you after agreeing with your initial wishes and plans. Too many women find themselves ensnared in a trap of dishonesty during their third trimester. "My doctor said she supported me having a natural birth on my first visit, but now she's saying I need a C-section because my hips are too narrow." "I always go postdates and my midwife was okay with that, but now she's saying I'll need to start discussing induction or transfer if I go past 40 weeks." "My OB was all for my VBAC, but now he's saying I can have a TOL (trial of labor) with restrictions during my labor and pushing." If your care provider no longer seems to be aligned with your philosophy and you've tried having an open discussion with them about it, that is no longer a supportive partnership. If your care provider initially agreed to your wishes but suddenly does not and is citing policies, restrictions, protocol, or any other excuse to justify their change in behavior that was not previously explained to you, there is one simple, yet powerful, thing you can do: fire your provider.

I switched care providers during this late stage of three of my pregnancies, and in talking to women all across the U.S. and internationally, I've found it's more common than you might think. Although it's certainly not what you want to be doing in your third trimester, many women find it to be an empowering decision in the end. One woman switched at 30 weeks because her OB told her she would only be able to push on her back and she knew she couldn't labor that way again. Another switched from one OB to another at 37 weeks to make sure she had the best chance at a VBAC—three unmedicated VBACs later, she knows it was the right decision. One woman told me she switched from an OB to a midwife practice at 29 weeks and was thrilled to no longer feel like a name on the schedule and to be looked at in the eye.

I spoke with a woman who switched care providers at 33 weeks when she felt her doctor became condescending and paternalistic. Seemingly out of nowhere, he began insisting she be induced at 39 weeks because she had risk factors for preeclampsia, and when she asked, he refused to consider additional monitoring as a course of action. So she switched to a doctor who respected her and her concerns. Her new care provider monitored her and she had an unmedicated birth at 42½ weeks. She never got preeclampsia.

I've known women who've fired their care providers while in labor, even at seven centimeters dilated! Or it can be for something seemingly simple and less dramatic: one woman switched at 30 weeks because although her OB was kind and knowledgeable, she just didn't connect with her.

If you're in your third trimester and you're planning a home or birthing center birth, making an appointment with someone who catches babies in a hospital, either a midwife or an OB, will help you have options should you need to transfer care at 42½ weeks. I hear this a lot, and it happened to me: at 42 weeks, a woman's home birth or birthing center midwife tells her she has to transfer to someone in a hospital. It really is best if there is some kind of backup care that doesn't put a woman who goes postdates in an incredibly stressful situation. That way when a woman hits 42 weeks, it's not this shocking "what's gonna happen" panicky time. Instead you transfer care to someone you've already met, who has you on file, and it doesn't have to be a traumatic experience. Everyone can still work together for a healthy outcome, mentally and physically.

I've seen this work beautifully in a Milwaukee birthing center—between their second and third trimester, all of the women in their care go in and have a visit with hospital midwives and OBs to meet them, see them, fill out paperwork, and even do an ultrasound. They tell women, "This question of transferring care will come up if you go past 41 weeks, and this is a chance for you to meet and talk with these hospital care providers about the possibilities if you need to go to the hospital to birth your baby." The independent birthing center midwives also transfer with their moms and stay on as support for their desired birth philosophy, making sure their voice isn't lost in the changes. I had that with my sixth when I chose to do co-care, and when I experienced it, I knew this is how it should have always been. This gives you options and support no matter what changes may occur.

Yes, we are dealing with the complicated subject of health care—specifically pregnancy and birth—with all of its rules and regulations and policies and practices, but you have no reason not to expect the same level of competency, care, and honesty from your care provider as you would expect hiring a care provider for a loved one. You deserve respect and care just as much as you think someone you care about deserves respect and care. It is up to you to set boundaries and teach others how to treat you in life, and this is no different. If your midwife or OB is not meeting the standards you set forth and they agreed to, then discontinue doing business with them and find another provider who will. You are worth it.

Self-Care During the Third Trimester

I've been saying this all along, but it bears repeating, especially as you near the end of your pregnancy: practice caring for yourself now so that you already have practice with self-care when baby comes. Self-care is a process. Put yourself in the mind-set and the habit of making sure you're taking care of yourself. When baby comes, everyone asks about the baby; no one is going to put you first but you. The first year you go into survival mode and that's okay; that's what it is. If you practice taking care of yourself during the third trimester and when preparing for postpartum, that helps you practice self-care while you're in survival mode, too.

Use self-care to help make decisions about labor and postpartum. For example, create boundaries around who you do or don't want in the birth room. This goes for everyone from your mother to your birth photographer, if you want to hire one. Be very intentional about whom you invite into your space. Worry about your own peace of mind more than you worry about hurting someone's feelings. Boundaries are self-care. It's okay to feel sad if your mother-in-law really wants to be in the room with you but you've asked her not to be—but don't feel guilty. She had her birth experience; this is yours. Some women give clear postpartum rules for visiting, too, including who or what comes into her home once baby is born. It's okay if you want to limit the amount of germs your newborn comes in contact with; it's just as okay if you want to limit the amount of extended family you'll come in contact with. Remember that you are part of your family, too. You wouldn't hesitate to protect your child, so don't hesitate to protect *you*—your physical, mental, and emotional health.

I'll talk more about postpartum self-care in part three, but for now here are some practical things you can do to prepare for postpartum: freeze meals, clean your house, and stock up on food gift cards. Hire a postpartum doula for a couple of nights. Put together a bin of essentials for baby *and* you: diapers, wipes, onesies, pacifier, and phone numbers of people to reach out to, snacks, water, and the Netflix remote. Have comfortable, stretchy clothes ready. And maybe some easy pampering things, too: face masks, bath soaks, essential oils.

You can prepare for your emotional health postpartum, too. Sure, prepping meals to freeze once baby comes is a brilliant idea, but who is the person you're going to call when you feel alone or overwhelmed? What are the one or two things you're going to do to remind yourself you're still you, even when you're sleep-deprived? We always say, "Reach out if you need help," and it's a lot more likely you'll reach out if you already have some people on speed dial (is speed dial still a thing?). Do you have a Snapchat buddy? A yoga teacher knowledgeable in postpartum physical and emotional support? A favorite Starbucks barista? These are wonderful lifelines for your postpartum. If it takes a village to raise a child, it also takes a village to support a parent. Just naming them is empowering. Let them know they're on your list, too; that you are going to need them in the months (and years) to come. Acknowledge to yourself that you are going through a time of transition, that birth and parenthood are unpredictable and beautiful and messy, and that every part of you will need time to heal, process, and find your new normal.

You can also prepare for birth and postpartum with sleep— guilt free. Get up ten minutes before everyone else (or stay up ten minutes after everyone else) and sit in some quiet place with coffee or carrot cake or whatever makes you feel happy. Do activities you loved before pregnancy. Exercise, whether that means taking a walk, dancing, doing some gentle stretches, or even a high-intensity, sweaty workout if that's something you've been doing before and during the first two trimesters. During my first pregnancy I went to a local pool almost every day, and I can't say enough about how much comfort it gave me, physically and emotionally. It was easy on my joints, soothed my muscles, and gave me a sense of deep relaxation while also allowing me to move around weightlessly during those last weeks of discomfort. Or you could take Epsom salt baths or long hot or cold showers. Listen to a soothing podcast. Get acupuncture. Have sex. Do nothing at all—guilt free.

I know some of you may not have a supportive partner or family nearby or any type of village. I know money may be tight. I know that the more tired you are, the more difficult it is to create and maintain boundaries, to clear your space of anyone or anything that's bringing in doubts, fears, or frustrations. I know because I've been there. But don't let any of those (or any other) valid reasons keep you from taking care of yourself in whatever ways you can that make sense for you. It's not selfish or extravagant to prioritize your well-being. Send anyone asking if you've had the baby yet to this website: www.haveyouhadthatbabyyet.com. There they'll get the answer loud and clear: unless you've seen a birth announcement, it's a big *nope*. In a world that gives you a lot of fear, anxiety, sadness, and doubt, I am giving you love. You are amazing. You are doing enough. You are completely worth it. You deserve peace. I'm giving you a moment to have it. Please accept it.

PARTNER POINT OF VIEW:
Guard Dog or Deer

At this point, your partner is nearing the end of her pregnancy. With your support, she has decided on a birth provider and location of the birth. She has most likely read numerous blogs and books on the experience of birth. The frequency of her prenatal appointments has increased and her provider is preparing her for what to expect from the birth process. The upcoming birth is consuming her thoughts nearly every hour, minute, and second of every day. She is more than ready to welcome a brand-new baby (or babies) into the world.

But are *you* ready?

If you are anything like me, you might be feeling some anxiety about the birth process. Your partner may have chosen to give birth with an OB/GYN or a CNM in the hospital, a midwife at a birthing center, or a water birth at home. No matter what scenario your partner desires, it will be a foreign experience for the both of you, whether it's your first baby or second, third, etc. The big difference for your partner is that she will be doing the work to birth the baby and her provider will be there to guide her through the process. You will be there by her side, encouraging and supporting her in the best way you can, based on the numerous discussions the two of you have had in the weeks and months leading up to the big moment. You are her safe space and her tether to staying focused and grounded.

But what if things go awry? What if, at the last moment, a perceived complication on the part of the provider arises and he or she veers off in the opposite direction from what was previously discussed? What if the doctor is pressuring your partner into having a cesarean because she isn't dilated enough according to their one-size-fits-all time line, or insisting on an episiotomy for no better reason than impatience? What if the midwife insists on stripping her membranes or begins pressuring her into taking Cytotec to induce labor before her body and the baby are ready?

The deer that wanders out onto a dark road, freezes when headlights approach, and ultimately gets hit by a car is never prepared for the dangers the road brings. Guard dogs, however, are always on alert and always prepared to defend their territory. It will be in those moments when your partner is being pressured into doing something that isn't in her best interests that you become the guard dog ready to fight tooth and nail for everything the two of you desire for the birth experience, or else you become the deer in the headlights who is paralyzed by the chaos that can ensue in the eleventh hour.

Surprisingly, your choice isn't made for you in the moment that a need arises. Your choice is made in the days, weeks, and months before your partner finally goes into labor. The choice is made when you attend all her prenatal appointments with her. The choice is made when you ask the provider any and all questions that arise in *your* mind. The choice is made when you do your own research online or read the books your partner reads. The choice is made when the two of you sit down to discuss the birth plan in detail and examine it from every angle together.

The former tennis star Arthur Ashe once gave his thoughts on what it takes to succeed: "One important key to success is self-confidence. An important key to self-confidence is preparation."

There are many factors that will go into the success of your partner's birth experience that are beyond your control. But being the one who will support her and look out for her best interests is completely up to you. When you are armed with the proper knowledge, you can go into the labor and birth with confidence that you can protect your partner's best interests when she will be at her most vulnerable. And anyone who attempts to tread on that vulnerability will back off when the guard dog makes his presence known.

PART TWO

. . . .

Options, Support, and Respect: Labor and Birth

*I do not care what kind of birth you have . . . a home birth,
scheduled cesarean, epidural hospital birth, or if you birth alone
in the woods next to a baby deer. I care that you have options,
that you are supported in your choices, and that you are
respected.*

You have made it past all the tests, questions, uncertainties, discomforts, and pesky comments of "When are you going to pop?" and "Are you sure there aren't twins in there?" And you haven't punched anyone. Tell me again why we don't get gold stars?

So, now what?

There are many factors that will affect your birth experiences in any setting, and in the following chapters I'll discuss the unique aspects of hospital birth, home birth, cesarean birth, and VBAC birth. I'll talk more about backup plans in chapter 8, but *no matter what kind of birth you're planning,* I encourage you to closely read the hospital birth chapter and fill out a hospital birth plan, because it's going to add information about things like birth classes and writing a birth plan philosophy—and it's better to be prepared and not use it than to not be prepared. If you're planning a hospital birth, I encourage you to read all the chapters, too! While all births are unique, there's good self-care and philosophy in each chapter and you never know what will impact you the most until you're in the moment. You may be laboring in the hospital and remember something you read in another chapter that you can pull from and focus on to help you bring your baby earth-side. Or you may remember something about care providers in the hospital chapter that supports you in your home birth. Don't skip over a chapter simply because you think it won't apply to you! There is wisdom to be gained from all births, and birth is unpredictable.

Chapter 4

Variations of Normal *Are* Normal: Hospital Birth Without Fear

....

*Birth is not a competition. We can celebrate and
support all birth experiences.*

Birthing in a hospital means you are bringing a human into the world in someone else's "house"—their rules, their policies—but your power is in *you*. Your power isn't in the hospital or the birthing center or the side of the road if that's where you birth your baby—the power is in you. Your body is your home, and you deserve to feel at ease at home. You matter in your birth experience and in your baby's birth story. Your feelings are valid. Your body is valid. Every single thing you do in your life—but specifically for right now I'm talking about pregnancy, birth, and postpartum—you should absolutely have a say in it. You can change your mind. You can use your voice. Your power is always in you.

You may be in someone's house during a hospital (or birthing center) birth, but during your labor, that hospital room is *your* space, your room. You can set the tone. When I went in to the hospital to birth my sixth baby, it was a last-minute unexpected change. I was planning a home birth, but ended up deciding to go to the hospital. As soon as I got into that room it was like a hurricane hit—people were running here and there, asking me to pee in a cup and change into this gown, sign paperwork, and a million other things. The mood was frantic and somber. Everyone there had a job to do and everyone was trying to check things off their lists and get their jobs done to get me ready for surgery. While I was in the bathroom changing into the hospital gown, I remembered one of my birth affirmations: "Don't forget to have a good time." And just like that, I could take a deep breath. When I came out into the room, I said, "I know that this is unexpected and this is not the birth I was planning, but today is still my baby's birthday, so can we please just smile and have a good time?" Almost immediately the whole tone and mood of everyone in that room changed. They were laughing and chatting and excited to celebrate this birth with us.

The point is, you get to decide how the vibe in your space is going to be. People will play off your tone and your energy. If you're combative and unsure, it's like you get a mirrored response. Don't start in that space. But if you go into that hospital saying, "I am strong, I am capable, and I want to have a great experience in this hospital," then you set the tone and energy of the space in a positive way. Once you've done that, if people don't want to get on board with you, that's when you rock the boat and start kicking people off your birth team or out of your birth space. But not before you define and create the energy yourself. Just by a simple statement or affirmation you can change the whole vibe—or at least you can figure out who's really on your team. That vibe is going to be different for every person and for every birth—for me, with that baby it was the mood that this doesn't have to be a bad thing just because my plans changed.

The majority of women in the United States birth in a hospital setting, so navigating the ins and outs and ups and downs of a hospital birth is key to creating the conditions for an empowered birth as opposed to a traumatic birth. I want women and birthing people to have a birth high, not birth trauma. Many women find their conversations in pregnancy with their care providers do not transfer over to the care they receive during labor or the experience they have when they birth. Or women go into labor when their doctor is not available and they get the doctor on call, a doctor they've never met before, or one with a wildly different philosophy than their own. As I listen to and read women's questions, frustrations, and birth stories within the Birth Without Fear community, one thing has become clear: many of the disappointments, hurt, and birth trauma are not due to where or how their baby came out, but are more directly related to how they were treated through labor, birth, and postpartum.

How do you set yourself up for the best possible birth experience, whatever that may be for you? I wish we could all move to Unicornilasia, where we birth babies through magic while we all enjoy sunny ocean days, tacos, and margaritas. That would certainly limit the amount of trauma you might experience. But assuming that's not happening anytime soon, here's my refrain: Know your provider. Know your hospital. Read birth stories. Learn from other's experiences. Know your options. Make a plan. Create a solid birth support team. Define the ambience of your space. Claim your power.

Care Providers

I can't reiterate enough that the person you hire as your care provider is significant for your birth experience. When you're in a hospital with its own policies and procedures, your care provider is your guide to how everything works. They have a relationship with the hospital you'll be birthing in, including many of the nurses and the hospital pediatricians. How they weigh decisions should the need for any interventions arise, how they speak to you and your partner when decisions need to be made, how much support they give, and what options they are willing to discuss are crucial pieces of your birth experience.

Speaking of pediatricians, after you have your baby, a hospital pediatrician will visit to look after your newborn. It's a good idea to have a conversation with your care provider or someone at the hospital about who the hospital pediatrician is and if you can have your own pediatrician come to the hospital, if desired (this usually depends on the hospital and state regulations). Schedule a call with whichever pediatrician will be used, and whatever your beliefs are, make sure your pediatrician is okay with that. It's much easier to have that conversation while your baby is still in your body than to have it for the first time when you are a very tired, new postpartum parent with a baby in your arms.

Issues such as the amount of skin-to-skin contact, wrapping the baby, rooming in (where baby stays with you instead of going to the nursery), as well as the use of vitamin K, silver nitrate, and the hepatitis B vaccine, are all things that may come up with the pediatrician or with your OB or midwife. I remember with my sixth baby, the pediatrician wanted to do my baby's footprints before they brought her to me! I said, "Um, I don't think her feet are going to grow much in the next hour, so you can wait, thank you very much!" As with all things, this relationship can be one of give-and-take—they can continue to monitor baby on your chest or put blankets over baby during skin-to-skin contact, for example, or you can kindly and calmly ask them to wait to take footprints and bathe baby until after you've had a chance to meet your baby and start bonding!

It also matters very much what kind of hospital you're birthing in. Is it a baby-friendly hospital?[6] If your hospital is designated "baby-friendly," it means they've undergone a rigorous process to make sure all their policies and procedures support parent and baby bonding as well as breastfeeding, which means that they are likely to be open to requests for skin-to-skin contact, delayed cord clamping, exclusive breastfeeding, rooming in, and gentle cesareans. You should also take a hospital tour sometime in your third trimester. That tour will give you the opportunity to ask questions about hospital policies and the hospital pediatrician, and to get a feel for the place. You should also be sure to have an ongoing discussion with your care provider about the hospital's policies and how they may affect your baby's birth.

With hospital births, many more possible interventions come into play. There are a lot of people coming into your space, monitoring you and your baby, and making suggestions or recommendations. This is good on the one hand, because you likely chose a hospital birth so that you'd have medical support close by, but it also raises questions: How do you determine when an intervention is necessary? How do decisions get made with so many voices involved (you, your support people, your care provider, nurses, and hospital policies)? It's important to keep in mind that interventions are not the problem per se, but rather how and why those interventions are introduced. There is a difference between an intervention that's introduced or suggested due to a true medical need—or even by your request—and one that's due to impatience; a difference between someone saying, "We're noticing this; let's discuss your options as well as our recommendations and reasons" and "We're noticing this, and you have to do this." In the first case, the care provider gives information and wants to talk options; in the second, the care provider uses fear and shaming to coerce the decision they want. Having a working, respectful, and good relationship with your provider can make all the difference here, but so can your clarity about this one thing: you deserve respect, options, and support. If you are feeling pressured into an intervention, if you are feeling guilted into an intervention, if you are feeling ignored, disrespected, or embarrassed in any way, as if you need to make a certain choice to please other people in the room, this is not good care and you deserve a second opinion—or a new care provider.

Know that although you are in someone else's house, you can request as many additional opinions as you desire. *Second opinions are normal.* And if they're okay (and even encouraged) with a dentist or a roofer, then they're okay (and sometimes recommended!) when it comes to birthing your baby. This includes wanting more information on a cesarean, an episiotomy, an epidural, and Pitocin, as well as the care of your baby once here. It's okay to switch care providers while in labor if at any point you don't feel supported. I know of women who have switched providers during labor—some as far along as seven centimeters dilated. It's probably not what you want to be doing at that time, but it really is okay. It happens, and I've never heard anyone say they made the wrong decision in doing it.

When we're talking about hospital birth, we also have to talk about labor and delivery nurses. Because here's the thing (and nobody really talks about this for some reason): no matter how much prep work you do to choose the best care provider for you, with a hospital birth, nurses make a huge difference in your experience. They are the ones typically sitting with and checking on you. You don't necessarily know these nurses beforehand, and it's pretty much the luck of the draw—while your care provider is on call and you will hopefully get them or their backup when you go into labor, you get whatever nurses are on shift during your labor. Just as with OBs, midwives, and doulas, there are really great nurses who understand variations of normal and respectful care and then there are nurses who simply do not. They are also human and all have their own comfort levels. If everyone is honest about their own philosophy, then we can all be matched up with nurses who align with us. We need to praise amazing labor and delivery nurses, but at the same time, know that if you don't get one who aligns with your birth philosophy you can ask for one who would be happy to support you.

Are your hospital nurses giving you supportive care or shameful care? You and your partner or your doula can be on the lookout for whether you have a supportive or unsupportive nurse and be prepared to ask if you want a change. This is another reason why having a doula is so great: if a nurse is scoffing at you because you don't want an epidural, or passive-aggressively saying, "Let me know when you change your mind," a doula or your partner can turn to you once you're alone in the room again and say, "Remember how we talked about you wanting a supportive nurse...it's okay to ask for another one."

It may be uncomfortable for a minute, but it's worth a few minutes of discomfort to have hours of labor with a supportive nurse. We're all so afraid to rock the boat, but, girl, you need to rock that boat so hard that it splashes anyone unsupportive out and they float back to shore, far, far away from you. Rock so hard that only the people who are going to hold on and are committed to being supportive and respectful of your choices get to stay in your boat.

Listen: nobody needs that shame. We can no longer allow this. If you don't feel comfortable asking for a different nurse (or midwife or doctor), have your mom, partner, doula, or whoever is on your support team to do it for you. They can be the bad guy. End of discussion. It can be that simple. If all it takes is a few minutes of discomfort to change nurses, do it. There is a wonderful nurse out there who would love to be part of your birth experience! No one else has to process and heal (physically and mentally) from your birth experience other than you. You matter. Your voice matters. Your support matters. Your experience matters.

Birth Classes

A lot of people take birth classes in preparation for birth and while I think they can be a good idea, it's important to keep in mind that just as with doulas, birth photographers, and care providers, much of it depends on who's teaching the class. You need to find the right fit for you.

Many hospitals offer birth classes you can take (usually for free or at minimal cost). I wouldn't recommend taking a hospital birth class as your only source of information because the people teaching those classes have their hands tied a little, based on hospital policies—they sort of have to say what the hospital tells them to say, you know? However, hospital birth classes can be good for helping you understand how that hospital works, so go ahead and take them if you want to and are able, keeping in mind the limitations that go along with them.

You may want to take a good pain management class like hypnobirthing so that you have a tool to help you cope with what labor is like—or you may want to read a book about it instead. No one ever said that you can only attend one type of class or conduct one kind of self-education! You can take one type of class, read a book on your own, and then chat with a friend to break down what each taught you—in other words, you can mix and match for what's right for you. The best birth education will empower you to understand your body in labor and to work with your body in practical ways. If you sign up for a class in which the teacher hands you a binder and proceeds to read the binder to you, take a different class. You can fire your birth class/teacher, just as you are allowed to switch providers. Remember to be loyal to you and your baby first.

Writing a Hospital Birth Plan Philosophy

The most empowering thing about a birth plan is not that everything on it is going to go exactly the way you want. The power is in the education that comes with creating one. Write your hospital birth plan with variations of normal in mind; for a hospital birth, your birth plan needs to be a little more open—you can have specifics and hard no's, but then other things can be open and more flexible. It's a philosophy as much as it is a plan—you want your plan to feel like "Here are some ideas, some things I am absolutely adamant about, some suggestions, and here is how I'd prefer to be treated, and how I'd like the experience to feel." In the end, whatever your birth plan and philosophy include, the most important thing is that you make sure your care provider is on board—and not just "on board," but supportive and encouraging of your wishes.

Create a simple but thorough document that clarifies for you and all the people who will be caring for you what your wishes and preferences are. You don't need to detail how you would handle every single potential scenario (is that even possible?), but instead you want to be really clear about how you'd like decision making handled.

Common topics addressed on hospital birth plans include how you would like to be touched (or not touched), your preference on some common hospital interventions, policies on transfers (if you're planning a home birth), and how you would like baby to be treated and his or her care handled. Here is an example, but you can change and add anything you'd like. You can write an extensive narrative or make up a simple chart.

HOSPITAL BIRTH PLAN TEMPLATE

Parent(s) Name(s):
Baby (boy/girl/surprise): [child's name]
Estimated Due Date:
Hospital: [location name]
Mother's Physician: [doctor's/midwife's name]
Doula:

I/We prefer the following during labor and delivery:

☐ A vaginal delivery over a cesarean.
☐ Membranes are not to be artificially ruptured.
☐ As few medications and/or medical interventions as necessary.
☐ Pain medication is not to be offered unless [mother's name] requests it.
☐ Saline lock (or hep-lock) to be used instead of a continuous IV.
☐ Freedom to move and choose position during labor and pushing stage.

- Use of intermittent fetal heart monitor (if continuous monitoring is *medically necessary*, a portable or wireless fetal heart monitor is preferred).
- Labor augmentation techniques are not to be used.
- No restrictions on [mother's name]'s urge to push.
- A local anesthetic to perineal area only if [mother's name] feels it is necessary.
- Risk tearing perineum instead of episiotomy.
- Natural delivery of the placenta.

I/We prefer the following immediately after delivery and postpartum:

- Skin-to-skin bonding with [child's name] immediately after birth.
- Initiation of breastfeeding as soon as possible after birth (if this is the mother's wish).
- Delayed clamping and cutting until umbilical cord has stopped pulsating.
- Allow [father's/partner's name] to cut the umbilical cord.
- Delayed newborn measurements, tests, and/or procedures until after sufficient skin-to-skin bonding and initial breastfeeding unless medical necessity dictates otherwise.
- No silver nitrate eye gel, vitamin K shot, or hepatitis B vaccine to be given to [child's name] immediately following birth without [mother's name]'s consent. If needed, [mother's name] will sign a waiver before surgery.
- [Child's name] is to be kept in room with [mother's name] at all times for the duration of hospital stay.
- All medical tests and/or procedures are to be done in room with [mother's name] and/or [father's/partner's name] present at *all* times.
- If [child's name] must go to the NICU due to medical necessity, [father's/partner's name] will be accompanying.

☐ If visitors arrive, please consult with [mother's name] and/or [father's/partner's name] before allowing them in the room.

☐ No pacifiers, artificial nipples, bottles, formula, or water are to be given to [child's name] for the duration of the hospital stay without [mother's name]'s and/or [father's/partner's name]'s consent.

Self-Care During Hospital Birth

Since you'll be birthing in someone else's "home," one of the best ways to practice self-care during your hospital birth is to make it YOUR SPACE. Decorate that hospital room. While you're there it's *your* room. Technically you're renting the room—you're paying for it one way or another. Bring battery candles—and use them! Dim the lights. If anyone needs to turn the lights on to do a test or check on you, say "okay," and turn them off again afterward. Don't ask permission, just flow with it. Bring affirmation cards on rings or laid out on a board. These can be as simple as big block letters that say: BREATHE, OPEN, and BRAVE; or longer sayings, such as two of my favorites: "Vaginas do open, babies do come out" and "Don't forget to have a good time." Or make a banner if you want to. Even if you never get the chance to look at them, they're there for your birth team to call out to you. Bring your own birthing gown, pillows, and blankets. Labor and deliver in your own clothes if you wish, and if anyone tells you can't, ask to see that policy in writing! Bring essential oils that soothe you. Have your favorite music put together in a birth playlist, or play hypnobirthing tracks, guided meditation, or even nature sounds. Or plug in a fan of some sort to create white noise. Maybe you want your special brand of toilet paper, your organic hand soap and lotion, or your favorite water bottle, lip balm, or comfy socks. Don't forget the hair ties!

Think about what makes you feel at ease and at home when

you are in your own space and try to re-create that. Now, you may not ever get to use these things if you have a very quick labor and delivery, for example; or you may find that those affirmations just annoy you in the heat of the moment, and that's okay. The details are less important than the intention to make this space yours. If none of these suggestions feel like you, that's okay too. They've helped you realize what is not for you and discern what *is* right for you. Be as at home as possible. Be you, do you.

But don't just bring a ball and candles, know how to use them—and if you don't, make sure you invite someone into your space who does. Someone smooth who knows just what to do and is like a godmother ninja, so you just look up and it's like, oh, all of a sudden here are these beautiful candles to help relax you through this contraction. Set it up yourself if you prefer. Sign someone up to be your check-in person instead of a doula or in addition to a doula, like those people at the water stations in a marathon. A friend or a support person whom you've asked in advance to go with you, get you settled in, and then leave. This does not need to be a commitment to being there throughout your whole labor. Every few hours they'll check in—even just with a text or a phone call—to make sure you have a good nurse and to see if you need food, batteries, or whatever. It doesn't have to be cut-and-dried, all-or-nothing, but you can be creative about what resources you want to pull together and how and when. If you expand your thinking, you can come up with ways to claim your space that work for you.

Get really clear about making it your space for your emotional and mental health, too. If you are separated from your baby's biological father, for example, you don't owe him or his mother space in the room, even though it's his child, too. We seem to be very into people being there the moment a baby is born these days, but you don't owe anyone entrance into your birth experience. If your brother-in-law invaded your privacy by coming in and out of your birthing room with your first baby, it's okay to have someone ask him not to come for your second birth. Or even better—don't tell them you're in labor. There's this sense of excitement when you go into labor, that feeling of "Here we go! It's beginning!" But labor and delivery, they're the last mile—when you literally have to shut everything else out, put on that last-mile music, and get your game face on. This is when you need to protect your space the most. If someone's feelings get hurt—well, sorry, but it's not their moment. It's yours. And remember that saying "It's easier to ask for forgiveness than permission"? That works here, too. If you need to be like, "Everything went too fast; I couldn't call..." then go right ahead and say that. Sometimes we just need to not create the drama ourselves, too. There is power in keeping things to yourself sometimes. There's power in not sharing everything. Sometimes silence is your way of keeping your power.

Think of yourself as assembling a psychological toolkit in addition to packing and preparing those physical items. Something I hear often is that women don't prepare for their psychological well-being in labor—either because you think trauma won't happen to you, or you put your trust completely in the medical system, or you think doulas or other kinds of birth support are only for more fringe, crunchy people. Sometimes it's because we think a care provider treating us in a way that feels uncomfortable or shaming is just normal medical treatment and there is nothing we can do about it. It's so easy to think, "Oh, this won't happen to me. I don't need to do the work of preparing myself physically or psychologically; I'll just let my care provider be in charge because I don't want to think about it." Most people don't spend much if any time in this world of labor and delivery—and what we know about it we learned from television and movies, which are notoriously unrealistic. I get it, I really do. Why would any of us even want to think about bad things happening to us? And why would we want to feel distrust for the people we are giving the responsibility to care for us? I don't want to scare you, and I know from experience that it's possible to have absolutely wonderful hospital birth experiences. But I also know that in order to give yourself the best possible chance of a healing or empowered hospital birth, you need to do the work to take good care of yourself.

All the prep work I've been talking about—doing your research, putting together a birth team, preparing and sharing your birth plan philosophy—are meant to help you focus on self-care during your hospital birth, rather than having confrontations and debating decisions in the moment. Prioritize things that will help your team care for you, and make it really clear to everyone how important that is to you.

You have power, even though it may seem at times as if everyone else has the upper hand. Give yourself permission ahead of time to ask for what you want, and also have the confidence and information to know that you can refuse something, ask for another opinion, fire your provider (or your doula), and kick people out of your space. If you're a people-pleaser or you know that you have a hard time creating and protecting your space or centering your voice, have somebody in there who gets it. When you're having a hospital birth, you have to know when to fight and when to ebb and flow.

What you really need is the freedom to go deep down inside yourself, without unwanted distractions, and with all the nonjudgmental support you can get. Self-care requires practice, practice, practice. And if there's any time to stand up for yourself and really ask for what you want, it's during labor and birth.

PARTNER POINT OF VIEW:
You Have a Voice

Everything is happening all at once.

If you hadn't done so already, you are frantically finishing packing a "hospital bag" with clothes, supplies, and snacks to take with you. You help your suddenly laboring partner into the car, toss the bag into the back seat, and leap into the driver's seat to get her to the hospital five minutes ago! You navigate the fine line between anchoring the gas pedal to the floorboard with your lead foot and not getting pulled over by a watchful police officer on your way to the hospital. You screech to a halt in front of the emergency room entrance and help your partner out of the car and to triage to get admitted immediately. Fearing a possible tow, you run back outside to legally park your car in the adjacent parking lot, grab the hospital bag from the back seat, then run back inside to catch up with your partner as she is being wheeled to labor and delivery, all while her contractions are strengthening and increasing in frequency. When she is taken to a room on the labor and delivery floor, you help her get her hospital gown on and settled into the bed as the nurse(s) strap her up to various monitors. The doctor—either the one you hired or the one on call—enters and assesses the situation before your partner is wheeled to the delivery room. Once inside the delivery room, you are instantly unsettled by the bright white LED lights, the frantic activity of the nurse(s), the businesslike detachment of the anesthesiologist, the annoying paperwork your laboring partner needs to sign for the administrative employee(s), and the gravity of the fact that you will have a new baby in a matter of moments or hours. Finally, the doctor returns, gloved up and ready to attend to your partner with instructions and pressure to induce labor or, if that doesn't fit the doctor's personal deadline, get prepped for a cesarean.

This is your cue to speak up on behalf of your partner. Her determination to follow through with the birth plan and philosophy she has voiced for months is subject to wavering amid her exhaustion and the chaos swirling around that delivery room. If it's a doctor she (and you) are not familiar with, he or she may be unreasonably insistent about following a rigid protocol with no validity outside of "hospital policy." Your partner might not have the necessary temerity to stand up to the doctor (and nurses, in some cases). You, however, do. In these instances when your partner's voice is either not heard, ignored, or seemingly overridden because she is the "patient" and not the doctor, your foremost task is to stand up for your partner and her physical and emotional well-being. She, more than ever, needs your voice.

The doctor and nurses on duty don't have to live with a lifetime of memories associated with this birth the way your partner does, or the way you do. This is how they earn a living for themselves. Your big day is just *another* day for them. They are providing a service that you are paying for (insurance or not), and your partner is entitled to receive the service she (and you) are paying for. If your voice is needed, use it. You can question every procedure and every decision. That is your right. If there are no complications and things are heading south for your partner due to the attitude of the doctor and/or nurse(s), speak up to steer things back on track. Again, that is your right.

If you and your partner found a doctor both of you trust and he or she is honoring your partner's wishes and/or birth plan, then things might be smooth enough that your own obstinacy on behalf of your partner is not needed, and you can simply focus on supporting the woman you love in birthing that new little addition to your family. If this is the case, congratulations on finding a great care provider!

On the other hand, if your partner is not being supported, respected, or given or allowed options by the attending birth team on duty, your voice can make all the difference in the world for your partner and your baby. Don't be afraid to use it.

Chapter 5

All Warriors Have Scars:
Cesarean Without Fear

. . . .

*Cesarean birth is birth. There are no "buts" or "ifs" when it
comes to which women deserve options, support, and respect.*

L et's kick this tired mind-set about cesarean births as only
being traumatic and disappointing to the curb: I'm here to
tell you that cesarean birth can be a powerful birth; it can
be a healing birth; it can be *a choice* for a healing birth. It's not
always an emergency, and even if it's your backup plan, it's still
birth. You don't have to automatically give up *anything* in terms of
options, support, respect, power, agency, and voice when you have
a cesarean birth. And the sooner we dispense with all the judgment and comparing, and acknowledge that all birth is birth, the
better.

Cesarean birth, like all birth, should involve informed choices
made with respect for your voice and feelings, and not decisions
based on fear or shame—and if fear is a factor because of the circumstances surrounding you, your baby, or your labor, then you
still deserve care given without shame, and you absolutely deserve
a lot of support through it. So much that we read about C-sections
is negative—and on some level I get that because I read all that

when I prepared for my VBACs—but it's okay to leave space for all of it: for cesareans to be empowering as a healing choice, a backup plan, or an absolute last resort. The world is not black and white. We just do the best we can with the information we are given in the situations in which we find ourselves. For so long I fought for a VBAC for myself, and then, when I least expected it, I found empowerment and healing in my last cesarean birth. I know that they can be powerful as well as disappointing and even traumatic, and I know that no matter what your experience with cesarean birth, you deserve the same options, support, and respect as you would with vaginal birth.

There are many ways to make surgical birth woman- and/or family-centered when that is wanted. If cesarean birth is your choice for a healing birth, then you already know it doesn't have to be a traumatic experience. If cesarean birth is not your first choice but you're prepared for one with a backup plan, then you're going to set yourself up to have a more family-centered or gentle cesarean birth experience if that possibility arises. If you've already had a C-section birth where you didn't have options, support, and respect, I see you and I understand if you have lingering hurt feelings to process, and even birth trauma.

We have some work to do to make sure unplanned surgical births are as inclusive and empowering as possible, for sure, just as we have work to do to make sure vaginal birth is empowering. Most of the things you read about C-sections are traumatic. You hear about disappointment, sadness, and shame. There are various reasons that cesarean births get the bad rap they do—for one thing, cesarean birth accounts for approximately one-third of all births in the United States each year, and there is a lot of questioning whether or not cesareans are medically necessary or just the preferred choice of your care provider.[7] U.S. cesarean rates rank quite high in the world: The Dominican Republic is the highest, with a rate of 56.4 per 100 live births, and the United States is not far behind at 32.8 cesareans for every 100 live births (New

Zealand's is 33.4 and Canada's is 27.1). Compared to countries with similar health care standards, like the United Kingdom, Sweden, Norway, and Spain, whose rates are among the lowest in the world (15–25 per 100 births), and given the World Health Organization's recommendation that a safe number of cesarean births would be limited to 10 percent of all births, you can see why there's concern.[8] There is also the concern that a cesarean means having your options taken away from you, losing agency over your body, and being denied your voice in your birth experience.

While it is important to try to change policies that limit options and women's voices, and I wish I could wave a magic wand and lower that number of cesarean births for the women who want it lowered, that can't happen overnight. I see this high number—30 percent—and I know it's a problem. I also know there are many people out there doing the work to change it. But, in the meantime, I want to make this kind of birth experience as good as possible for mom, baby, partner, and family. While we work to enact change over time, let's also work on lessening birth trauma and promoting empowerment. It doesn't have to be either-or. I want to be part of the solution, and certainly part of the solution is education and lowering the number of unnecessary C-sections. The other part is making sure necessary and wanted C-sections are not traumatic.

I'm holding space for you if you want to have a cesarean, or had one and didn't want to and are dealing with that. If you had a traumatic cesarean birth, I hear you. If you are afraid you may have one and you're not quite sure how best to prepare for it, read on.

I remember discussing the cesarean birth of my sixth baby with my friend while I was in recovery. Processing is so natural and healing. I had called our birth photographer to tell her that I'd had the baby via C-section, so we would not be doing birth photography. She told me she was sorry. It was a natural reaction, but I remember thinking, "I do not want that to be the reaction every time I tell someone how this baby was born." My friend who was with me said, "This is *her* birth story, J, and that's okay." She was right! Her birth was not and never has been a disappointment! It was the right birth for this baby.

Because here's the thing: cesareans don't have to be this shameful experience that nobody wants to talk about. Since they do account for so many births, let's not ignore them; instead, let's limit the trauma they may cause by helping make family-centered cesarean practices the norm, not the exception. Everything I've been saying all along about how powerful and capable you are, how wise your body and your baby are, how you deserve individualized care without shame—all of that remains true if you have a cesarean birth. In fact, surgical birth is quite amazing in its own right, and it requires its own kind of strength, love, and healing. I want to radically shift the faulty thinking that sometimes accompanies C-section births from one of disappointment to one of empowerment.

My hope for cesarean births is that they are fully supported and joyful birth experiences, decided upon with complete trust in your care providers and absolute respect for your voice. If you do have a traumatic experience, then you deserve the space to process everything you're feeling. If you choose one because that is the most healing option for you, your baby, and your family, then you deserve to talk about that baby's birth story with happiness and pride. And if you end up needing a cesarean as a backup plan, you deserve to have a say in that experience and to feel cared for without shame. Remember that you deserve individualized care as well as care informed by best practices—you and your baby are unique.

Planned, Last-Minute Planned, and Emergency Cesareans Without Fear

There are different ways you may have a cesarean birth experience: planned from the beginning; a change of plans—sometime between getting the positive test and your due date, the need or desire arises to change to a cesarean birth; and an emergency change of plans, which usually occurs after you were already going through labor—this was never part of the plan, and then at some point it becomes part of your plan. If you planned your cesarean birth from the beginning, you will certainly want to have a cesarean birth plan in place, one that answers the question: What does an empowered cesarean birth look like for me? In the second and third instances, additional questions arise: What does an empowered backup cesarean birth look like for me? What do I keep from my (original) plan when going into survival mode? How do I process that change?

This is why it's good to have a cesarean birth plan from the beginning, no matter what your ideal birth experience may be. Whether it's a discussion in labor or leading up to labor, it's wonderful to be able to say to your care provider, "We talked about this before, let's go over this again"; or, "This is what we said we wanted; is this what we still want? It's been a while since we discussed it." Perhaps you decide to plan an induction because your partner is only home from the military for a limited time, for example. In this case, you'll have some time to plan, but probably not much; and if you have a C-section birth plan in place, it won't be the first time you're having this discussion with your care provider and birth team.

If you end up in an emergency C-section situation, birth plans more often than not go out the window, but if you have a cesarean birth plan in place, little things will be remembered. You, your birth team, and your care provider will do what all of you can to maintain parts of that plan, and it can take some of the shock out of it. I always make the distinction between a traumatic event and trauma—an emergency cesarean might be a traumatic event, but it doesn't have to turn into birth trauma if you have good support, if your doula is there supporting you, if your OB is there for you, and if once you're in your recovery room you've got a strong team there to support you, and to hold your hand as you process.

So write a cesarean birth plan philosophy, and in the writing of it, ask yourself what would make for the best possible experience for you and your family. Just as importantly, creating this plan will give you the opportunity to ask your care provider whatever questions or concerns you may have about cesarean birth. Don't let it just be something you hope won't happen, with fingers crossed and eyes shut tight to the possibility. Plan for the unplanned so that you give future you the gift of space, honesty, and support around this decision.

Writing a Cesarean Birth Plan Philosophy

Whether you're planning a cesarean birth or only considering a cesarean as a backup plan—and whether you plan to birth in a hospital or in the woods over a frolicking stream—I highly suggest that you have a cesarean birth plan and philosophy, just in case. Sometimes, due to the fast and surgical nature of a cesarean, doctors and hospitals forget to include the family, and especially the mother, in the birth. A cesarean is a birth, and needs to be treated as one. If you are in the position of needing a cesarean, please know that you can still make choices in your birth and have the birth you desire. It may feel that with a surgical birth you give your body and your baby's birth over to the surgeon and other care providers, but that does not have to be the case. Birth, like life, is unpredictable, but you can still have an empowering experience if you go in with knowledge and not fear—or if you go in with a little fear, also with your voice and a lot of support.

More and more hospitals and care providers are getting hip to family-centered cesareans, and even if your care provider or hospital hasn't, that doesn't mean you can't ask for one. When I say "family-centered cesarean"—also called a "woman-centered" or "gentle" cesarean—I'm referring to a whole group of options that will help you and your birth team feel less like you're undergoing the cold, disembodied procedural surgeries of decades past and more like you're having the joyful, interactive birth experience you may desire. A family-centered C-section often means things like skin-to-skin bonding; a mother-centered C-section usually means being scrubbed in and helping birth your baby.

In a cesarean birth plan, you may want to ask that your care provider explain the surgery to you as it happens. Since it is surgery as well as your baby's birth, you may want to explore the possibilities for minimal sedatives after birth (which may help you feel as awake as possible), the options for being up and walking as soon as possible after surgery, and how quickly you'd like your catheter and IV removed.

If you'd like to, go ahead and ask that the screen or drape be lowered just before baby is born, and that the surgery is performed slowly (you can also request a clear drape, although many hospitals in the United States still don't allow a clear drape, so you may have to fight if that's important to you); gentle, slow contact by the surgeon as baby is born, rather than grasping and quickly pulling baby out; allowing eye contact between mother and baby as baby is passively and/or actively born; and, if possible, allowing the cord to continue pulsing after the birth so baby can start breathing on his or her own while still attached to the placenta. Ask to see and touch the placenta and cord if you'd like, and to see and touch anything that will help you feel as connected as possible to your body and your baby.

You can also request skin-to-skin contact immediately or soon after birth, as long as you and baby are well. If you are having a hard time holding your baby due to being numb or possibly having the shakes from medications and surgery, then there's an opportunity for your partner to experience skin-to-skin contact and start bonding. Other things you may want to ask for: immediate breastfeeding, if desired; a warm blanket during surgery if possible; for the surgeon to reinforce your uterus and use dissolvable stitches for closing—that is, double-suture your uterus (a double layer is often wanted for a VBAC) and suture on the outside instead of using staples.

Consider your recovery and the moments after baby's birth when writing this birth plan as well: Would you like to keep baby with you at all times once you're back in your recovery room? Would you like to keep visitors out of your recovery space? Would you like baby's bath to be delayed rather than given right away? Will you be nursing on demand? Here's a Cesearean Birth Plan Template that you can use as you start to name and discuss your wishes with your health care provider.

CESAREAN BIRTH PLAN TEMPLATE

Parent(s) Name(s):
Baby (boy/girl/surprise): [child's name]
Estimated Due Date:
Hospital: [location name]
Mother's Physician: [doctor's name]

I/We prefer the following during surgery:

☐ Only use medications suitable for breastfeeding.

☐ If possible, provide a non-drowsy, anti-nausea medication.

☐ Explain the surgery to [mother's name] as it is being performed.

☐ Provide a warm blanket during the surgery.

☐ Provide a clear screen so [mother's name] may view the birth. If a clear screen is not possible, lower the screen just before the delivery so [mother's name] may view the birth.

☐ Perform surgery slowly enough to allow baby to breathe on his or her own while the umbilical cord continues to pulsate.

I/We prefer the following immediately after delivery and in recovery:

☐ No sedatives are to be given after the birth so [mother's name] can be alert and attentive during [child's name]'s first day of life.

☐ Double-suture the uterus with dissolvable stitches and suture external layers instead of using staples.

☐ Facilitate skin-to-skin bonding with [child's name] immediately after birth. If not possible, [father's/partner's name] will bond skin-to-skin with the baby.

☐ Initiate breastfeeding as soon as possible after birth unless medical necessity dictates otherwise.

☐ Allow [father's/partner's name] to cut the umbilical cord.

☐ Newborn measurements, tests, and/or procedures are to be delayed until after sufficient skin-to-skin bonding and initial breastfeeding, unless medical necessity dictates otherwise.

☐ No silver nitrate eye gel, vitamin K shot, or hepatitis B vaccine is to be given to [child's name] immediately following birth without [mother's name]'s consent. If needed, [mother's name] will sign a waiver before surgery.

☐ When [mother's name] has been cleared as stable and taken to a recovery room, she and [father's/partner's name] would like to be left alone to breastfeed [child's name] in a peaceful environment.

☐ [Mother's name] would like a snack or meal and to have IV removed as soon as possible following surgery.

☐ [Mother's name] will be nursing [child's name] often in order to stimulate production of breastmilk and soothe baby.

☐ [Child's name] is to be kept in room with [mother's name] at all times for the duration of the hospital stay.

☐ All medical tests and/or procedures are to be done in room with [mother's name] and/or [father's/partner's name] present at *all* times.

- [ ] [Child's name]'s bath is to be delayed until the evening following birth.
- [ ] If [child's name] must go to the NICU (neonatal intensive care unit) due to medical necessity, [father's/partner's name] will be accompanying.
- [ ] Remove [mother's name]'s catheter the evening or morning after surgery.
- [ ] [Mother's name] will be up and walking as soon as possible.
- [ ] If visitors arrive, please consult with [mother's name] and/or [father's/partner's name] before allowing them in the room.
- [ ] No pacifiers, artificial nipples, bottles, formula, or water are to be given to [child's name] for the duration of the hospital stay without [mother's name]'s and/or [father's/partner's name]'s consent.

Talking With Your Care Provider

A cesarean is still your baby's birth and your birth experience, so you want to make sure you and your provider are on the same wavelength. Even if you're not planning a cesarean birth—even if you're not planning a *hospital* birth—talk to your care provider about a C-section so that you're not blindsided. I know that if a C-section is not wanted, it can feel better not to talk about it at all because you don't want to even consider the possibility; or that it can be easier to just feel open to it but not really prepare for it. But making the switch to a cesarean birth is not just changing plans; it's adding surgery into your plan and really changing the dynamic of your birth and postpartum—new care providers may become involved or more involved, the location of your birth experience will change, new questions and forms will be introduced, and your healing will be different as well. In other words, it's kind of a big deal. You can't plan for every possible thing. Birth is unpredictable. But you can take some time to talk with your care provider about what a cesarean birth might look like for you so that you have options.

Some good additional questions to ask while interviewing care providers: If all is well with myself and baby, can we schedule the birth on or after my due date? What happens if I want to or I do go into labor before the scheduled cesarean? You may want to wait until as close to the due date as possible or until your body starts very early labor. Some women will want to wait until they go into labor to know their body and their baby are ready, or at least go postdates. The most important thing is listening to your intuition about it.

Also, talk to your doctor about different pain med options. What are their thoughts on epidural versus spinal anesthesia? What are my options for screen (clear screen)? When will I first see my baby? Where is the warmer and pediatric team located in the OR? I'd like it to be within my vision; is that possible? Once baby has been checked on and cleared, I would like to have skin-to-skin contact and/or establish breastfeeding (if wanted). What kind of incision and suturing will you be doing? The thinking behind this conversation with your providers is the same as it's always been: Are you receiving care without shame? Are you being respected? Are you receiving individualized care? Does this relationship feel like one based on trust and mutual philosophies? Are you on the same page? There's no wrong question. Any other question your beautiful mind comes up with, ask.

In addition to talking with your care provider, you can educate and prepare yourself by doing things like watching videos of natural cesareans to normalize and make sense of some of these options.

Self-Care During a Cesarean Birth

The most powerful thing you can give yourself for self-care with birth is space: space to feel how you feel if you *want* this type of birth without fear; and space for if it happens to be the birth your baby needs, even if it was not part of your plan.

When we talk about skin-to-skin bonding, specifically with surgery, it releases hormones and it really does help. Brandon and I both had colds when our sixth baby was born. When I was moved to the recovery room after surgery, we took turns holding the baby for extended periods of time because the oxytocin literally revived us from our achy, lethargic stupors. I can still picture Brandon groaning in disappointment every time I requested the baby back.

I know it can be very painful when things don't go as planned, and you may have additional feelings to process in the event of a surgical birth. But when things don't go as planned, remember that it's not *our* birth, it's our baby's birth. It's our experience, but it's their birth. We don't have all the say; there's another human being who has a say in this.

If your birth is different than you planned, that will take emotional energy to process. With an unplanned surgical birth, your postpartum will be different than you planned—not just your emotional healing but your physical healing, too, will be different. You'll be healing from being pregnant, healing from surgery, and on top of that your boobs will hurt. There is so much time needed to heal. But you *will* heal. You just need to allow yourself the space.

PARTNER POINT OF VIEW:
Being Exponentially Supportive

Labor and birth are a time of uncertainty for the partner. We like to find solutions, fix the problems, and keep an overall eye open for when we are needed for solutions and fixing. If a problem arises during labor or birth, we can't fix the problem. If our partner elects to have a cesarean ahead of time, there is little we can do control the situation if that is what is called for based on the circumstances of health or personal choice. The only power we have in the event of a cesarean is of the supportive kind, and it is during this time that our support must increase exponentially.

Think about it. The woman you love has carried a growing baby in her womb for somewhere between nine and ten months. She has endured aches, pains, hormonal changes, rearranging of organs, excessive fatigue, shortness of breath, poor sleep, a weak bladder, and the list goes on and on. Now, she is in the operating room, receiving anesthesia to numb her from the chest down while the OB and nurses are prepping themselves for the impending cesarean. When the doctor begins the surgery, he or she will cut through skin, subcutaneous tissue, fascia, multiple layers of muscle, more fascia, the abdominal wall, and then the uterus to finally reach in and pull your baby up and into the world for the first time.

Your partner will be incapacitated on the operating table and looking to you for comfort during the operation and immediately after. Yes, the doctor and nurses will communicate with her about the surgery and the baby, but you will be the one she will trust most. You've been by her side for this whole journey, validating her choices and taking up the slack in areas she couldn't because of the rigors associated with pregnancy. It is you who has the most invested in her well-being and the well-being of your baby, and it is you who will need to reassure her every step of the way once the baby has arrived. From removing fluid from the lungs and checking limbs and digits and hip joints, to weighing and measuring and the Apgar test, she will want to know everything that is happening to her brand-new baby. It will be essential that you ease her mind by informing her of what is happening, if she cannot see for herself, and that you listen to her, *really listen*, for what she's saying she needs—either with her words or in her actions.

In the hours, days, weeks, and months ahead, she will need you even more. Her body will need time to heal from the operation. Movement of every kind will be slow and filled with soreness. If your home has stairs, she will need your steady hand to help her up. She may need help off the couch or the bed. If your partner is breastfeeding, she will need you to get up out of bed in the middle of the night to hand her the baby. Expect to be the one to carry that baby in his or her car seat, exclusively and indefinitely.

In your work to support your partner, don't forget to consider yourself. If you have family who can come over and help, never turn them down. You will need to rest as well, and some much-needed breaks given by close family members or friends can be just the recharge you will need. If you don't have support nearby, consider a postpartum doula who can be there at night to assist your partner with the baby while you sleep. This is an invaluable option for you if you are feeling worn down and weary, especially if you already have one or more kids to care for. Your partner absolutely needs to rest and recover, but so do you.

And at the end of the day, don't forget to remind yourself that this is all temporary. Your partner will heal from her cesarean as time goes on, and your family will find a new ebb and flow together in time.

Chapter 6

Vaginas Do Open, Babies Do Come Out: VBAC Without Fear

. . . .

You wonder how much longer you can do this. You can't feel the baby's head yet. You have no choice but to be in the moment. Then, just when you can't, you do. Transition of a woman in birth, motherhood, and life.

I'm going to be completely real with you: if you want to birth your child vaginally after previously having had a C-section (a process known, as we've discussed previously, as a VBAC), you will probably have to fight for it. But I will also tell you this: you are strong and you are capable. Believe in your cervix. Believe in you. Feel absolute conviction in your goal to have a vaginal birth.

When it comes to VBACs, we've come a long way but we have so much further to go. "You'll never be able to have a home birth," my OB/GYN told me as she operated on me during my second cesarean birth. Can you just hold space for me for a moment? Because that's not just a bad bedside manner, it's bad human decency. There I was: over 42 weeks' pregnant, after three days of labor and now in the hospital, numb, exhausted, being cut open in a cold OR, completely vulnerable, and my care provider was judging me, my body, my future pregnancies, and births.

I looked at her and said, "Can we discuss this later?" It was all I could think to say in the moment. Let me hold space for you, too: it is all too common for women wanting a vaginal birth after cesarean to have to fight an uphill battle—in my case that battle started before my cesarean had even ended—against misinformation, stigma, and just straight-up doubt from those with medical authority.

Know that you will fight for this not just for you, but for your children and for future generations. Women have been fighting for rights over their bodies and lives since we came into existence. It can be disappointing when we have to fight to use our voices or to be heard or to have a say over our birth experience. But you are in a long, long line of generations of women before you who had to do the same. You will need to fight not only "the system" but also your own inner voice and fears, your own internalized doubts and insecurities. You will need to be in a very strong mental place. You will need to fight to find peace and a belief in your ability to birth this baby out of your vagina. We owe it to the women who went before us, to our daughters, and to ourselves, to fight for this.

The fact that you're willing to go through what you're going through—that makes you amazing. This is not about VBACs versus cesarean births. Birth is not a competition. This is specifically for women who have a desire for this type of birth and need to be held up by the strong voices of those who have been in their shoes.

VBAC is its own category distinct from vaginal birth—not just statistically but mentally. Because when you're fighting for your VBAC, you're already a parent. You have a child but you've never given birth vaginally—and that can be hard to wrap your mind around. When you birth this baby, even though you're a mom, it's like you're a first-time birthing mom—probably with some emotional baggage on top. It's a lot to work through. And so a VBAC birth requires its own energy and its own preparations; it will bring up its own questions, concerns, and fears. It is different, and we can and should honor that.

When a hospital puts a VBAC ban into effect or an OB practice doesn't support women in planning for a VBAC, they're taking away your options. Removing options is never the answer. Taking an option away from a woman regarding her body, her autonomy, her pregnancy, and her birth—it's wrong. I understand that these hospitals and practices think they're doing a good thing, but all they're really doing is backing women into a corner—and that corner, it should be said, when banning VBACs or not supporting VBACs, is surgery. We have become so desensitized to the fact that we're asking a woman to have surgery. Surgery is not without its own problems and risks. If they're trying to make it safer by taking the option and possibility of vaginal birth away but actually making it *less* safe by forcing women to have surgery, then this "no VBAC" edict is actually counterproductive. All it's going to do is create more problems. Why is it so hard to support women? Crawl up out of there, unsupportive providers. My vagina didn't ask for your permission. My cervix never said, "Hey, is it cool with you, hospital, if I have this baby this way?" It's really weird the restrictions we try to put on women's bodies, especially the cervix and vagina.

But sometimes the doubt doesn't come from the hospital or your care provider; it comes from within. Questions like "Is something wrong with me?" or "Am I crazy to even try this?" can plague women who want to try for a VBAC. The truth is that the facts support success for VBACs. But in order to make this part of your birth journey, you'll need an extra boost of information, support, and positivity. It takes every ounce of mental strength to birth a baby vaginally after one or more cesareans. The last thing a birthing mother needs is opposition from her providers or herself.

All this talk about goddesses and queens, but are we really treating ourselves and each other that way? Where's the care provider who says, "Wow, she has worked so hard, she has mentally prepared, physically prepared to open and birth this baby, and somewhere along the line she was failed, so we need to lift her up while she goes through this experience"? *That's* treating a woman like a goddess and a queen. Not "Well, you're a VBAC, you're overweight, you go postdates; what's wrong with you?" The moment when a woman feels like she's failing—*that's* when you treat her like a goddess. When she's suffering and having a hard time, *that's* when you treat her like a queen. If no one else will believe in you, I will. Draw on those generations of women before you who fought, and for the generations to come who will look to you to see what you did. That fighting spirit in you should be *more* reason for your birth team to cheer and support you, rather than a reason to judge and shame you.

VBAC Birth Plan Philosophy

Your VBAC birth plan philosophy will be much like a hospital birth plan and/or a home birth plan if you're hoping to birth at home. However, if you're a VBAC mama, you may want to be extra intentional about creating space for yourself in your birth plan philosophy, because you already have one or more surgical births in your history and now you're fighting really hard for a different kind of experience. You may be bringing additional fears and anxieties into your VBAC. You may be struggling with how to handle expectations, doubts, and hopes. You may very adamantly not want anyone in your space to even mention the word "cesarean" unless it's truly a medical emergency. And you can make space for any of these or other concerns in your birth plan. If you write this into your birth philosophy—for example, if you have PTSD from a previous surgical birth and you'll need extra space to make decisions or process feelings—that lets everyone on your birth team and everyone who will be caring for you in labor and birth know how best to support you. A VBAC birth plan philosophy is not the space to avoid previous births; it's the place to make space for everything you've learned about yourself from them.

VBAC-Friendly Provider

If you can find a VBAC-friendly provider, that means you will have to fight less. Check with your local ICAN (International Cesarean Awareness Network) group to get recommendations for care providers supportive of VBACs. If you are using a doula, ask them for recommendations—actually, even if you're not using a doula, go ahead and call one up and ask them for a list of their top three care providers. Don't be afraid to ask around: to call doulas, midwifery practices, and friends and family who've had babies in the past few years. We need to do this work to create little networks of empowering, women-centered care providers in our own cities and towns.

With birth comes uncertainty. Birth is unpredictable. All you can do is look at your body, your history, and your experience and come up with an individualized care plan with your provider. When talking to your care provider about a VBAC, you may want to know: Are they willing to talk about what your pregnancy looks like, how your baby responds to labor, and how your body handles it all? You may want to ask, "What are my chances and why? What are my risks and why? What's in my favor and why?" This conversation should be an evaluation of those risks and possibilities among yourself and your providers. You want someone who will say, Let's look at these numbers, let's look at you, and then let's come up with a plan for you.

What if—and this happens to so many women—you think you have a VBAC-friendly provider and then you get to 36-plus weeks and suddenly scheduling a cesarean is brought up, completely throwing you off your mental preparation? Or if your care provider starts talking about giving you a "trial of labor" (TOL) in which they have you labor under the supervision of an OB with restrictions and limits to determine your chances of having a successful vaginal birth? Or if you're told by your provider suddenly at some point in the process that you will have to be hooked up to IVs and can't change positions, after you expressed a different preference and thought you were on the same page? This is why it's so vital to have a provider and team 100 percent on board with *your* plan. If a straightforward conversation about this doesn't feel productive, changing providers is always an option.

And what if you can't find a VBAC-friendly provider? What if you live in an area that isn't VBAC-supportive? Build a really strong birth team. Hire a doula—or two. Make sure you have a friend or partner who is completely on your team. Have people you can bounce ideas off. If you have to travel to a supportive OB or hospital—that's okay, do it! I've known women who've traveled three hours to a supportive care provider. They feel (and I agree) that it's that important. I know a woman who rented a hotel room across the street from a hospital for her home birth, because her home wasn't close enough to a hospital and she wanted to be able to move quickly and easily if necessary. Sometimes, when options are taken away, you have to get creative. Look at your own situation and see what works for you.

Now, if VBAC poses true concerns for the health of you and your baby, that is different. Never lose sight of your intuition, even if it's telling you something you may not want to hear.

Self-Care with VBAC

VBACs require an extra dose of fierceness because you're not just going for a vaginal birth, you're going for a vaginal birth with a history that could work against you; you want to make damn sure no one's negativity or doubt creeps into your space. So let me put it in all caps: MAKE YOUR BUBBLE. Say to yourself: the only people who can be in this bubble are people who believe in my ability to birth this baby out of my vagina. Strongly protect your mental space.

But there's a part two to this fierce attitude: I call it "fierce as f*ck but being reasonable." In other words, part of planning a VBAC is a kind of single-mindedness about your birth experience—that nothing's going to stop you from birthing this baby from your vagina. You need that "Yes, I can!" attitude. You need to put on your loudest pump-me-up music, pull on your (virtual) boxing gloves, and give yourself and everyone around you a riveting locker room speech about overcoming adversity—or whatever type of metaphor works for you. As a result, VBAC women can get a little intense and single-minded because you become a woman on a mission. I know you need that passion. For the sake of your own self-care, though, be strong, but never lose sight of your intuition.

If you do end up needing a C-section, it's okay. It's okay if you end up making that choice for yourself, or if not. It does happen: you plan and work, and yes, even obsess for nine to ten months, and BAM! Life reminds you we only have so much control. You may be at peace with that. You may not find peace about it for some time. Both are okay. You're allowed to change your mind at any time. You're allowed to be disappointed and hurt if things don't go as planned. Life is unpredictable. Make sure you have people around who have unwavering belief in your ability to birth your baby vaginally *and* who know that if everything needs to change, it will be okay. It's still your voice, and you still deserve to be heard.

Remember that ICAN chapter you checked out when looking for a VBAC-friendly provider? They also have support for CBACs (cesarean birth after cesarean, or a cesarean birth despite working toward a VBAC). Help and support are out there. You are not alone. Your emotional needs are valid and you deserve the space to process and heal.

PARTNER POINT OF VIEW:
Support Equals Confidence

A VBAC is a big undertaking, perhaps the biggest undertaking of your partner's life. Pregnancy already requires so much emotionally, but the asterisk a VBAC adds to your partner's history can be an emotional uphill climb. However, you have the power to support her all the way to the top of that climb.

As a husband of a VBA2C (vaginal birth after two cesareans) mom, I would be lying if I said I didn't worry at least a little bit with each of January's three vaginal births. When the control is out of our hands as partners, a certain level of worry or anxiety is par for the course. And when even the slightest chance of a severe complication exists for a VBAC, however small it may be, it does truly add another layer of trepidation for those of us supporting a VBAC mom.

The key here is twofold: (1) assure your partner as often as necessary that her body *can* do this, and that *she* can do this, through your words and actions; and (2) trust in your partner's ability to have a vaginal birth *despite* a prior cesarean.

If your partner has done her due diligence and hired the best care provider to suit her needs throughout the pregnancy, labor, and birth, you can rest assured knowing someone is being paid to know what to do in case the pregnancy and/or the birth encounters a medical complication of some sort.

Your focus will be on the support your partner will need during the long months of pregnancy and how you can positively affect the outcome of a VBAC through that support. It doesn't matter if your partner has hired the most spectacular doctor or midwife to see her throughout the pregnancy and attend her birth, she has or will get push-back from someone—whether it's raised eyebrows and a polite (or impolite) decline from another professional during her initial search, uninformed concern from a friend, or ignorant pressure from family. If your partner is having doubts (and she will), don't feed her uncertainty with your own worries. Instead, lift her up with your support—through words and actions. Remember, your first task is assuring her early and often that her body *can* do this, that *she* can do this. Take the little one(s) out to the park for a couple of hours so she can have silence to read, think, and focus on her VBAC. She will need all the rest she can get going into the VBAC, so get up with the kids on your days off so she can sleep in. If she is tired and achy, run her a bath or give her a massage, or both! If she wants to employ the help of alternative health care providers to add another layer of confidence in her body, accompany her to the chiropractor, acupuncturist, and/or naturopath to show your support. If you have your own questions and concerns (and you will), go with her to every prenatal appointment and bring them up to the doctor or midwife. Maybe the answer you get isn't just something you need to hear, but something your partner needs to hear as well.

By looking at every situation with a supportive eye and responding with a supportive action, a funny thing will happen along the way: your own worries and anxiety will lessen and your confidence in your partner and her pregnant body will increase. Think of it as a positive feedback loop. Confidence in your partner and her pregnant body will blossom and grow when you take supportive actions that help her develop confidence in herself and her pregnant body to see a VBAC through to its happy end.

Hands-on training works because we learn by doing. Faith in the pregnancy and birth to happen as it naturally should, from you and your partner, requires consistent support from *you*. Don't underestimate the power your support and belief will have on the success of her VBAC. In fact, use that power often and wisely.

Chapter 7

Everything You Ever Wanted to Know About Home Birth But Were Afraid to Ask: Home Birth Without Fear

· ·

I knew my body could birth a baby the way millions of babies had been birthed before me, and I came to realize that the only person who believed I could without doubt was me.

I f home birth is what feels right to you, I'm here to tell you: you can do this. When everyone's telling you can't, I'm telling you you can. Many, many women before you have birthed their babies without a hospital. In their own homes. Probably women in your own family not that far removed from you. Ignore everyone who's telling you you can't do this. You can. When some stranger in line at the grocery checkout chides, "You're going to wish for an epidural," or when your favorite aunt admonishes you over the dinner table, "That's not safe," let me be the voice you hear that says: you can do this.

Maybe you *will* wish for an epidural, but what does that person who brought that negativity into your life know about your body and your baby and your journey? Everyone has an opinion. When your plan is anything even remotely against the norm, you're going to get a lot of comments. I know it gets exhausting hearing everyone judge you all the time. Make your bubble. It doesn't mean putting your head in the sand; it means saying, "I am aware. I am not ignoring risks. I am more aware of my risks than you are. I have done and continue to do my homework about this. If you can't deal with it, walk away. Out of my bubble."

We need more honest, unbiased conversation happening around home birth. I have a secret to tell you: we can empower ourselves through educating ourselves and we can make decisions based on information and intuition instead of based on fear. There is a lot of fear and misconception about home birth. A lot of people see it as an extreme choice, something only crunchy, off-the-grid, anti-modern-medicine families do. There is also a misunderstanding that those who want them are completely in the know about them, and everyone else is afraid to ask. But the truth is, there is not a lot of good, open, unbiased conversation going on about home birth. Home birth is an option—one among others—and we should treat it the same way, because you deserve to have your questions answered without shame or judgment.

If you've ever wondered about home birth or had questions, you deserve to explore all the potential ways to have a home birth that works for you and your family. There are variations of normal with home birth, just as with all birth. I don't tell people how or where to birth. I just want all birthing people to know they *do* have options and that they deserve respect and support through this journey.

Home birth can be a beautiful and wonderful option. It's comforting to be in your own space, without people putting you on a time limit, without the sound of beeping machines, and with no one touching you when you don't want to be touched, no one coming in and out, turning on the lights, interrupting your birth space. Your labor-land mind-set should not be unnecessarily interrupted. There is a natural flow to labor and birth (mentally and biologically) and we want that to be respected and honored, not constantly interrupted with doubts and checks and unwanted intervention suggestions. The familiarity of laboring and birthing at home can offer a feeling of peace to you and your partner. You have complete control over who is in your space in home birth, while in a hospital you just don't.

With a home birth you also shouldn't have to fight as much if you have the right midwives and birth team surrounding you. You get to invite in only people who make you feel empowered and proud—people who support you. I'm not saying you can't make this happen with a hospital birth; however, you are not in somebody else's home or territory, so you can feel like you're truly in charge. Because you are. For some people that's really important, for some people it's not. A birth without fear, an empowered birth, will be different for every person. Some women feel safer birthing in a hospital. Some women feel safer birthing at home. It is not a competition, and we can feel how we do for ourselves while respecting others who are on a different journey than our own.

For me, home birth was the only place I could have the space where all the people in the room believed in me. I didn't want to ask permission to do basic things like eat and walk around. I also didn't want anyone interrupting our bonding with baby. In my experience, the biggest relief was that after our baby was born, in our own space, only the tests we wanted done were done, and no one was interfering as we got to know our baby. My other children woke up to find Brandon and me relaxing on the couch in the living room, and they all came in close to meet their baby sister. It was the most empowering experience, not just because of the healing birth, but because of how our postpartum began as a family of six.

Home birth is a safe option for many women, but it does come with its own set of questions, concerns, and plans to make. If you're curious about home birth but you're afraid to bring it up—or if you have brought it up and are getting judgment from friends and family—here is the honest and open conversation you've been looking for. I want to empower you by giving you the information on why people choose home birth and answering questions that you're not going to find everywhere else.

You might find after reading all this information and all these chapters that laboring at home close to transition and then transferring to a hospital for the birth is the way for you. Maybe after reading all this you decide, *Nope, I want a hospital birth.* And maybe you have had one (or more) hospital births and then decide you want to go for a home birth. There is no one way or right way; you, your care provider, and your birth team are the only ones who can know, based on you, your health, and your baby's health, what is best for you and your baby. No shame. No judgment. Just love.

If you do decide a hospital birth is right for you, that doesn't mean all this information is useless—with the right providers you can come close enough to creating this home birth feeling in a hospital birth if that's where you need to be. You can have a beautiful hospital or birthing center birth. Even if you don't want a home birth, the questions and ideas here can inspire you to create a comfortable, empowering, or even healing hospital birth.

And if what you really want deep down is to home birth—let's do this.

Variations of Normal in Home Birth

I want to answer some of the most common questions I hear about home birth, to help demystify it and to empower you to make the best choice for you and your baby. If you want more information on any of these issues, discuss them with your care providers.

Water birth at home: Why do I see so many? What's it all about?

Some women choose to labor in a tub or the shower because the water helps with pain relief and easing their way through transition. Note that you may have this option in a hospital or birthing center as well, so go ahead and ask around in case you end up transferring or if you're planning a hospital birth.

Some women choose not only to labor in water but also to birth their babies in water, because they believe birthing in water is a gentler transition from womb to vaginal canal to earth. In my experience, laboring in water close to and during transition is very good for easing pain, but I like to feel grounded and on land during birth and there's an instinctual part of me that doesn't like water birth, so I only use the tub before I start pushing.

The most important thing to keep in mind is that water birth doesn't have to be all or nothing. It's an option. It can be great, but you certainly don't have to do it, and if your instincts are telling you otherwise, then don't worry about forcing it. If at some point you want to get yourself under some running water or sit in your tub during your home birth, then go ahead and give it a try. If birthing in water is something that interests you, make sure you discuss ahead of time with your care provider how they make sure baby is safe during water birth.

Where do you get the tub?

Some midwives have a birth tub they will bring, or you can rent a birth tub, use your own tub, or buy a kiddie pool.

How do you keep the water warm? How do you empty it afterward?

These are things your birth team will do—your husband, partner, doula, and midwife will help with setting up and filling the tub, keeping it warm by adding hot water as needed if necessary (a midwife's tub may be heated), and emptying it—usually by taking a hose and letting it drain outside (it's good for your plants!).

Do baby and I need to check in at the hospital for any reason afterward? Can I have a home birth and stop in at a hospital for any needed tests—or even for a day or two of bonding with the help and support of nursing staff? Who checks on baby's and my health in the first few days after birth? Who follows up?

Your midwives can do everything they do at the hospital if mom and baby are both healthy and well. They are perfectly capable of doing all the newborn exams and doing stitches on mom. In some states midwives can give Pitocin if needed. It's a synthetic oxytocin, used to help the uterus contract during labor and/or to control post-birth bleeding. If there is anything going on with mom or baby, you can absolutely go to the hospital after birth. Transfers aren't just an option during birth; you can transfer postpartum. Do you need to? Absolutely not. Most people just go to their pediatrician a few days after baby is born, or the midwife comes back a few days after birth to do follow-up exams, PKU tests, etc. But if anything comes up or you want to transfer to a hospital for any reason at any time, you can.

As for a day or two of bonding with the help and support of nursing staff—all I can say is, wouldn't that be nice? I wish we had that kind of postpartum care! You can hire a postpartum doula or other support to come in and give you some extra help in those first few days, but otherwise, unfortunately, no. A hospital won't check you in after home birth unless there is a physical need (unless something is wrong).

What about birth certificates and other "official" documentation like social security number?

Your midwife submits all that paperwork.

Can I have a home birth if I'm having twins? What kind of high-risk situations affect my ability to have a home birth?

Questions of high-risk pregnancies and home birth depend on state laws—the question isn't really "Is it legal for me to birth my baby at home?" but, according to state laws, "Is it legal for a midwife to attend my birth at home?" For twins, breech, and VBAC, among other high-risk situations, you will need to find out if it's legal for a midwife to attend. And if it is legal, you need to have that discussion with your care provider about what your risks are and what things you're going to do to support your unique situation. In the case of twins, for example, there should be additional midwives attending.

Is it safe? Can midwives handle things like postpartum hemorrhaging, if baby isn't breathing, if I need stitches, if there's meconium, if I need Rh shots? What happens if something goes wrong?

All birth and pregnancy come with risk, and these are absolutely important questions to ask the midwives you interview. In terms of what care midwives offer, a lot depends on the state—but, in general, yes, midwives are trained to handle things like postpartum hemorrhage, if babies aren't breathing, and other situations. If something goes wrong, you will transfer to a hospital. Part of good midwife care means knowing when to transfer.

What happens if I'm planning a home birth and I go into labor early, before 37 weeks?

If you go into labor before 37 weeks, you have to transfer to a hospital—and that's because of concerns about things like lung development and the fact that your baby may need to spend some time in the NICU, so you want quick access to that support.

How do you handle pain management during a home birth?

In a home birth, pain management is up to you and your partner and your doula more than your midwives. You will not have access to an epidural with home birth. However, there are some things you can do to cope with pain. In addition to laboring in water (tub and/or shower), there are coping techniques you can look into, like swaying your hips, moaning, using heating pads and/or cool cloths, and trying different positions. For me, I found that leaning over and sticking my hips out and moaning helped me manage.

This is a good conversation to have with your doula, so that she can remind you to do hip squeezes, horse lips, moaning, and more. You can also ask your midwife if they have access to a TNS machine (electrical currents that can soothe your nerves) and laughing gas. They may have other suggestions about different techniques they've seen mamas get help and relief from.

How is routine prenatal care handled with a home birth— things like ultrasounds and lab tests?

Many midwife groups do all the prenatal care right there in their offices. Some things—like listening to heart tones with a fetoscope or Doppler—they can do in your home, but ultrasounds need to be done somewhere else, so if they don't have their own office space for this, they'll send you to an office that they work with. Lab tests can be done in a midwife's office or in your home, and then they'll be sent out to a lab.

What about the mess? In the bathtub, on my bed, anywhere? What about the smell? Do I have to sanitize everything? Who cleans up and how? Will I ruin my mattress?

Your birth team will clean that all up while you're bonding with your baby. It's pretty awesome. I recommend layering a sheet over a mattress pad and then another sheet over a second mattress pad. That way you can easily remove a layer or two until everything is more under control and you are no longer bleeding. Layering is a good idea in general: if you rent and have wall-to-wall carpets, for example, have some chucks pads (bed pads) ready to throw around on the floor.

Birth doesn't leave a lingering smell.

You don't have to sanitize yourself from yourself. In a hospital you're around other people's germs, but at home it's just you. If you cut your finger you don't sanitize the whole house, right?

What about the sound, for women who live in apartments or in cities with lots of neighbors?

Both of my home births were in two-bedroom apartments with tiny bathrooms, and no one heard me. With my first home birth I did let my neighbor know, but they didn't hear anything anyway. Oftentimes, women tend to labor at night when everyone is sleeping, and no one is awake to be bothered. If you're in touch with your neighbors you can give them a heads-up, but they probably won't hear—or they'll just think you're having amazing sex.

Questions and concerns about sound, smell, and mess are all good questions, and I find them very interesting because they seem to stem from the prevailing medical philosophy of birth that we've all been socialized on: that birth is dirty, loud, scary, messy, and, well, weird. But it's not weird. In fact, it's very normal and common. It's no louder (or messier!) than a party you might host. You don't have to apologize for your body. You don't have to be afraid of its sounds and smells and movements.

Will my dog or cat freak out?

This comes down to knowing your pet—if they are clingy and nasty with others, or just anxious in general, it is probably a good idea to put them out in a yard or make arrangements for them to be somewhere else safe. Creating your birth space includes who you let into it. If a pet has a stressed-out vibe, then just like with an anxious human, they should be kept out of your space. Most pets are pretty chill about birth, though—it's an animal experience, after all, and it's not such a big deal for them. I've seen some beautiful photos of little doula dogs patiently and gently attending birthing women.

Where do I give birth? What if I have a really small house? What if I rent?

That's going to be different for everyone. Listen to your instincts. If you need to squat, squat. If you're tired but you need to squat, squat on the toilet. If you need to be in the dark in an enclosed space, go there. You don't need a whole lot of space to be on your knees and moaning or squatting or pushing. When you give birth in a hospital, you're in a hospital room, and that's not a very big space. And in a hospital there can be a dozen people coming in and out of that small space, with all kinds of big monitors and machines and whatnot. But home birth is intimate, small, just for you. You don't need a lot of space. If you need to, make a corner that's for you—clean and nice with the vibe and energy you want for your birth. And tell everyone in your house not to touch that area, not to make it dirty.

I could be wrong, but I'm assuming there's nothing in your renter's lease that says you can't give birth in your apartment. Just have someone on your birth team lay down pads so you don't stain the rug if you're renting.

How much does it cost?

If there was ever a variation of normal answer, this would be it. The cost for birth in general and the cost of home birth in particular vary so much. It depends on the state or country you live in, your insurance, and the midwife. The best advice I can give you is to ask around.

Care Provider

Midwives are the provider of choice for nearly all home births, so choosing the best midwife for you is key for a home birth.[9] While there are many excellent midwives, the same care in choosing a provider should be taken as when choosing an OB/GYN.

We need to have an honest conversation about hiring midwives. I have to be real with you: not all midwives are created equally. I thought they were, and it put me in a situation of mismanaged care, not being supported emotionally or physically, and a transfer that ended in a repeat cesarean. Am I blaming the midwife? Yes, mostly. It is her profession, and she completely misread and mismanaged the care. What could I have done differently, and what was my responsibility in it? I could have asked more questions of other home birthers in the area, as well as of the midwife. I could have educated myself further on the variations of midwifery care, which depends on the midwives themselves and the credentials they hold. I had to learn from this experience and take the new knowledge with me into my next experience. That is how we gain wisdom. It's what we do with those experiences and information moving forward that matter.

And because of that experience, I'm willing to say it: sometimes midwives are not great. But they *can* be great. They can be absolutely wonderful. I think women are afraid that if they speak up when a midwife gives unsupportive advice or shames a woman or makes her feel uncomfortable or unsafe that they will be ostracized from their communities. The truth is, we need to be willing to talk about our experiences. We need to hold midwives just as accountable as we hold OBs.

Being a home birth midwife is hard work. There's a fine line between giving the woman space and options, and also making sure they're having a safe birth, and I don't think that's for the faint of heart. Being a home birth midwife takes strength and competence. You need someone who values safety over their ego. You need a levelheaded midwife, and she needs competent, levelheaded backup, because being a midwife is exhausting. You need someone who knows when you need more and when to transfer you to a hospital.

So when it comes to hiring a home birth midwife, just as with all care providers, you need to interview them and their backup or support team. Thoroughly. Maybe even more thoroughly than you would your hospital or birthing center care provider. I've said it before and I'll keep saying it: who you bring into your birth space matters. Just as there is a variation in care with OBs, there's going to be a variation of care with midwives.

There are different kinds of midwives: a licensed professional midwife (LPM), a certified professional midwife (CPM), and a certified nurse-midwife (CNM), with the last being the highest level of training. Again, a lot comes down to state laws and what level of education they require midwives to have, as well as to what education the midwife wants. It's okay to ask: What's your level of training? How many years of experience do you have? What are your maternal and infant outcomes? But also keep in mind that it's not merely the letters they carry behind their name but who they are as a person. Just as with OBs, notice how they treat the people they care for, and how they treat spouses and partners.

Additional questions you may want to ask at-home midwives include: What emergency equipment do you bring and when do you set it up (immediately, so that it's available if needed)? How many trained people will you have with you? What is your training and experience? How do you monitor baby and me after birth? What are your transfer rates and how do you handle transfer? Part of safe midwifery care is knowing when to transfer. For those of us who are fighting hard to have a home birth VBAC, that can be a hard pill to swallow, but put on objective goggles about transfer rates. Ask why those women were transferred. It's not just the rate or number of transfers that matters. There's a difference between transferring because this midwife wasn't supporting home birth and doing so because she knows when to call for a transfer—she knows when safety and health are at risk. Consider the following: How close are you to the hospital? How feasible is good backup care?

Pain Management

One of the biggest concerns with home birth is how to deal with pain—fear can arise when you know you don't have access to an epidural if you should decide you want one. Know that you can transfer if you decide you need that pain medication. But also spend time before labor processing what to do with pain when it comes.

The reality is, you're going to feel pain. Your body and your life are opening up to birth a human. No matter how this baby comes out, you're going to feel pain at some point. You don't get an epidural postpartum (if only!). You can't avoid it, and you can't tiptoe around it. See it as part of the transition process. Prepare yourself to work through it. Something for you to think about in the weeks leading up to birth: what will help soothe you, what to do with pain. Don't ignore it; make space for it.

Self-Care During Home Birth

You are allowed to change your mind without shame. Again: you are allowed to change your mind. Give yourself the space to do so. Right now. Give yourself permission to change your mind at any time during this journey. When my friend's partner got his wisdom teeth pulled out, at first he said he didn't need any extra pain medication. When he changed his mind an hour later, asking for the pain medication, she didn't say to him, "But you said you didn't want it before—what happened? Are you too weak to go without it?" No. She simply understood that his need changed, that he wanted different care, and she gave him the meds. Why is it so different for women? Why is it that if we say we want an unmedicated birth and then we decide we need something to ease the pain, we are made to feel shame and failure? Or if we want a home birth and then decide a hospital feels better? And that can go both ways—maybe you're planning a home birth but no one you know ever has and they're judging you, or you normally identify as a natural, crunchy mama so your friends are judging you for wanting to birth in a hospital. Stop trying to fit a label or meet an expectation. Do you. And YOU are allowed to grow and change.

We can't allow that shame into our birth space or our lives. We have to honor what feels right to us as women. We know. You know where it feels safe, where it feels right, and how to listen to that intuition even when nobody else understands. This goes for listening when it changes, too. Do not justify your why, but instead demand respectful care and your absolute right to change your mind. You can be an incredibly intuitive person no matter where and how you birth. You don't have to be birthing near a waterfall under a rainbow to be in touch with your intuition. Sometimes you just need space.

This needs to be said when it comes to home birth self-care: just because you have an all-natural home birth in water does not mean that you're going to be okay with every single thing that happens throughout your labor and your birth. It also doesn't mean you won't have postpartum depression or other postpartum mental and physical health challenges. If you need to say, "I'm not okay that I wasn't listened to," or "I don't like how my cervical lip was handled," or "My doula or midwife didn't hold space for me," then give yourself the space for that honesty. Home birth can be beautiful, soothing, and, in my experience, an empowering and healing birth, but if there are things that don't feel right to you, you still get to say that. You still get to own your feelings and process your experience in a space of love and support.

HOME BIRTH PLAN TEMPLATE

Parent(s) Name(s):
Baby (boy/girl/surprise): [child's name]
Estimated Due Date:
Midwife (Team, if applicable): [midwife's name, assistant midwife's name]
Doula: [doula's name]
Other Support People: [birth photographer, friends, family, caregiver for siblings]

I/We prefer the following during labor and birth:

☐ Environment to be regulated according to [mother's name]'s preferences, such as conversations and noises kept to a minimum, lights dimmed or off, specific music or playlist to be played, water kept to a comfortable temperature range in birthing tub (if applicable), specific essential oils to be diffused, etc.

☐ No mention or discussion of time unless [mother's name] asks.

☐ To be left alone with [father's/partner's name] when requested.

☐ Cervical checks kept to a minimum and done only when deemed medically necessary by [midwife's name] and consented to by [mother's name].

☐ [Mother's name] is GBS-positive and [consents/does not consent] to chlorhexidine wash during labor.

☐ [Mother's name] is GBS-positive and [consents/does not consent] to antibiotics (at early labor/when water breaks).

☐ Use of (Doppler/fetoscope) for intermittent fetal monitoring.

☐ Monitoring of [mother's name]'s vitals to be kept to a minimum unless [midwife's name] deems it medically necessary.

☐ Recommendations to ease labor, such as breathing techniques, pain relief, hot and/or cold compresses, etc.

☐ Healthy snack suggestions and reminders to stay hydrated to maintain [mother's name]'s energy.

☐ Frequent checking in and encouragement during labor.

☐ Freedom to move and choose position during labor and pushing stage.

☐ Suggestions and/or help to guide pushing if needed.

☐ [Midwife's name] to [give/not give] perineal support and/or massage during labor.

- ☐ [Mother's name] or [father's/partner's name] to catch the baby if requested.
- ☐ Birth photographer to be present to take pictures (if applicable).
- ☐ No one else present during labor without [mother's name]'s consent.

I/We prefer the following immediately after birth and postpartum:

- ☐ Skin-to-skin bonding with [child's name] immediately after birth.
- ☐ [Mother's name] or [husband/partner's name] to announce the gender if it's unknown.
- ☐ Initiation of breastfeeding as soon as possible after birth (if this is the mother's wish).
- ☐ Natural delivery of the placenta, no managed third stage of labor or cord traction, unless intervention is medically necessary for safety of [mother's name].
- ☐ Delayed clamping and cutting until umbilical cord has stopped pulsating.
- ☐ Allow [father's/partner's name] to cut the umbilical cord or do cord burning if preferred.
- ☐ Delayed newborn measurements and tests until after sufficient skin-to-skin bonding and initial breastfeeding, unless medical necessity dictates otherwise.
- ☐ No silver nitrate eye gel or vitamin K shot to be given to [child's name] immediately following birth without [mother's name]'s consent. Discuss delay or alternatives.
- ☐ [Child's name] is to be kept with [mother's name] at all times.

Note: If a hospital transfer is necessary, please refer to the hospital birth plan in chapter 4. If a C-section is needed after transferring to the hospital, please refer to the cesarean birth plan in chapter 5.

Provider Self-Care

This is true for all care providers, but I want to say it loud and clear in particular when it comes to at-home care providers who won't necessarily have the backup that those in a hospital setting do: birth workers, from doulas to nurses to midwives to OBs, need to practice self-care. All birth workers need to practice self-care. If you have an exhausted, strained, worn-out provider, they are more likely to make decisions or say things that are unsafe or unsupportive. In a home birth, if a midwife is exhausted and she's the only one with you, or if your midwife is strained because she's pregnant or postpartum herself, that is not practicing good self-care. It is vital that we create and expect a culture of self-care not only for pregnant and postpartum people and their families but for care providers, too.

If you are a birth worker and reading this, I want to say this: I know that it's a hard profession—and it's a hard profession to practice self-care in. It's hard to get enough sleep, to set enough boundaries. I know as care providers you want to support your patients and give them the care you know they deserve, but don't forget about you. You have to take time off. Choose sleep. Say no. Set boundaries. Accept help. Birth workers need to practice self-care before preaching it.

And so, as the person birthing, you can ask it of your provider: Are you too tired? What do you do for yourself? What backup support will you have? These are all good questions to ask, both for your own information and because it humanizes your provider.

Birthing Centers versus Home Birth

Some women wanting something in between a home birth and a hospital birth will opt for a birthing center birth. Birthing centers vary, but in general they are set up with the idea of a home in mind yet in close proximity to medical care. Some feel very homey; others feel more like a small, intimate hospital.

As with all things, there are great birthing centers and not-so-great birthing centers. They also vary a lot in terms of their relationship to hospitals, the kind of care providers they have on staff, and even the vibe in the space: some birthing centers are a lot more laid-back and homey, while others are a more comfortable option within a hospital-type setting. You need to do your due diligence and collect information about the individual birthing center and the midwives (and sometimes the overseeing OBs) who will care for you and your baby.

A lot of the variation in birthing centers (and birth options in general) comes down to state laws, so look into your state laws and just as with home birth midwives and OBs, consult and interview different practices. There are a few additional questions you may want to ask when interviewing birthing center providers. For example, is it certified professional midwife (CPM) based or certified nurse-midwife (CNM) based? A certified professional midwife (CPM) is a midwife who has met the certification requirements of the North American Registry of Midwives (NARM) by serving as an apprentice to a proficient midwife or graduating from an accredited midwifery school or program, both of which require completing the entry-level portfolio evaluation process. A certified nurse-midwife is a registered nurse who has completed a graduate-level nurse-midwife program accredited by the Accreditation Commission for Midwifery Education (ACME) and passed the certification exam administered by the American Midwifery Certification Board. Other kinds of midwives to look for are certified midwives (CMs), who will have completed a graduate-level midwife program accredited by ACME and passed the certification exam administered by the American Midwifery Certification Board; and lay midwives (LMs), uncertified or unlicensed midwives whose training usually consists of an apprenticeship or self-study.

Are they supportive of vaginal and unmedicated out-of-hospital birth? What are their transfer rates? How do they handle transferring? Why do their transfers happen? And what are the outcomes? If I transfer, will my midwife stay with and support me through the changed birth experience? Will I still have supported postpartum care? Will I have the same midwife the whole time, or are you on a call schedule? Do you have OBs who oversee the practice?

Also keep in mind that birthing centers will often have more restrictions than home birth and hospital birth. You may be "risked out" based on your BMI, your history of going postdates, and your history of C-sections and VBACs. Again, this likely depends on state laws as well as the views and capabilities of the midwives or the OB, or hospital policies.

BIRTHING CENTER BIRTH PLAN TEMPLATE

Parent(s) Name(s):
Baby (boy/girl/surprise): [child's name]
Estimated Due Date:
Birthing Center: [location name]
Mother's Midwife: [midwife's name]
Doula:

I/We prefer the following during labor and delivery:

☐ Membranes are not to be artificially ruptured.
☐ As few medications and/or medical interventions as necessary.
☐ Pain medication is not to be offered unless [mother's name] requests it.
☐ Saline lock (or hep-lock) to be used instead of a continuous IV, if an IV is deemed necessary.
☐ Freedom to move and choose position during labor and pushing stage.
☐ Use of intermittent fetal heart monitor (if continuous monitoring is *medically necessary*, a portable or wireless fetal heart monitor is preferred).

- ☐ Labor augmentation techniques are not to be used.
- ☐ No restrictions on [mother's name]'s urge to push.
- ☐ A local anesthetic to perineal area only if [mother's name] feels it is necessary.
- ☐ Risk tearing perineum instead of episiotomy.
- ☐ Natural delivery of the placenta.

I/We prefer the following immediately after delivery and postpartum:

- ☐ Skin-to-skin bonding with [child's name] immediately after birth.
- ☐ Initiation of breastfeeding as soon as possible after birth (if this is the mother's wish).
- ☐ Clamping and cutting umbilical cord delayed until it has stopped pulsating.
- ☐ Allow [father's/partner's name] to cut the umbilical cord.
- ☐ Newborn measurements, tests, and/or procedures to be delayed until after sufficient skin-to-skin bonding and initial breastfeeding, unless medical necessity dictates otherwise.
- ☐ No silver nitrate eye gel or vitamin K shot to be given to [child's name] immediately following birth without [mother's name]'s consent. If needed, [mother's name] will sign the waiver before the surgery.
- ☐ [Child's name] is to be kept in room with [mother's name] at all times for the duration of the birthing center stay.
- ☐ All medical tests and/or procedures are to be done in room with [mother's name] and/or [father's/partner's name] present at *all* times.
- ☐ If visitors arrive, please consult with [mother's name] and/or [father's/partner's name] before allowing them in the room.
- ☐ No pacifiers, artificial nipples, bottles, formula, or water are to be given to [child's name] for the duration of the birthing center stay without [mother's name]'s and/or [father's/partner's name]'s consent.

PARTNER POINT OF VIEW:
What I Wish I Had Known About Home Birth

I classify the birth of our fourth child, our first successful home birth, as the best day of my life. I was so proud of January. I was so excited to get to know the latest addition to our family in the comfort of my own home, on my own couch. Nothing has compared to it before or since.

A home birth is a completely different experience than a hospital birth, with the potential to be the best experience of *your* life, too. Missing are the bright white overhead lights, bustling nurses with monitors and testing devices in hand, emotionless anesthesiologists with eyes glued to vitals, concerned doctors impatiently wondering if they will need to induce or perform a cesarean, administrative employees inconveniently needing signatures, and the horrid cafeteria food drowned in butter or grease or both. What you have instead is the comfort, peace, and familiarity of your own home. Sure, there will be birthing supplies like chucks pads, receiving blankets, extra towels, and washcloths lying around in plain sight that you normally wouldn't have. There might be a big birthing tub that you'll need to set up right in the middle of your living room or bedroom. If you hired a midwife, she and her assistant will be around for the birth. Maybe a doula, too. But all of it, everything and everyone, will be in *your* home.

In a hospital setting, your partner will need you to be on constant alert to see that her wishes are being respected and her needs met. If you are lucky enough to have a supportive hospital staff on duty, you might be able to let your guard down. If the hospital staff is repeatedly pushing this intervention and that test, it can leave you exhausted and worn out.

At home, you and your partner have full autonomy over the situation. You don't have to stand up for her and be a guard dog. You don't have to worry about being a deer in the headlights either. Your level of involvement in the birth of your child is up to *you*, not hospital policy. You are at *home*. Of course, it is wise to listen to the birth professionals you have hired and follow their recommendations. But, in the end, you and your partner have the final say over every situation. If there is an unnecessary recommendation or intervention that your partner doesn't agree with, she can refuse without needing to sign a waiver that she is going against medical advice. She is at *home*.

On the other hand, complications do arise and it is important to know that and be prepared—just in case. January attempted a home birth with our second child that became a hospital transfer when her labor extended to a third day. We weren't prepared for that scenario, and the bombardment of panic and stress we encountered by that hospital staff left both of us emotionally reeling for months afterward.

It is important to remember that, as much as you and your partner prepare for the home birth, you should have a contingency plan in place in case a hospital transfer becomes a medical necessity. Meet with your midwife's backup doctor and learn his or her philosophy and mind-set on labor and delivery. Hopefully, your home birth turns out as perfect as you and your partner have planned, and you never need to utilize that doctor's expertise. But it's better to cover all of your bases in case an unforeseen situation *does* arise, so you and your partner won't be caught unawares. It took us until January's last pregnancy to put this plan into action, but it gave her, *and* me, peace of mind knowing that she could birth our sixth baby at home or in the hospital and she would be supported either way.

With the home birth of our fourth child, we knew that if a complication did arise, we were only a five-minute drive from a nearby hospital. But there were no complications. Instead, January labored in the quiet of our home once the older kids fell asleep. When she felt the need, she labored in the bathtub, not worrying if her care providers would "let" her. When labor progressed into transition, she got out of the tub and into a squatting position to birth the baby, not on her back in a hospital bed with her feet in stirrups. January gave birth moments later and I was there to catch our new baby, not deliver her. When the baby took her first breath and cried out, I handed our new arrival over and hugging my exhausted wife, crying, "You did it!" without nurses and doctors interrupting to perform newborn tests and measurements. January dozed as she nursed the baby to sleep in *our* bed a short time afterward, and not worrying about hospital staff intruding on her privacy the moment she closed her eyes. Later that morning, our kids woke up to their brand-new sister with ear-to-ear grins. It was a momentous, joyous, surreal, and most of all, peaceful experience.

It can be for you, too.

Chapter 8

When Your Destination Requires
a Detour: Backup Plans Without Fear

*Life rarely goes as planned. Birth is one of the most unpredictable
experiences you will have. Prepare and prepare some more, then
surrender to the journey.*

You have read everything you can find, researched every
type of birth and outcome, spoken with family and friends,
interviewed care providers, consulted with your midwife
and/or OB at every checkup, and made a plan—and that's beautiful and empowering work. Through all of this planning and learning there's one thing we have to remember: when it comes down
to it, birth is unpredictable.

So what happens when you think your baby's head is down,
ready to engage your pelvis and exit the womb in the final weeks of
pregnancy, but instead you find out that your baby is breech? What
happens when you plan and visualize a home birth for ten months,
but end up being three days in labor with a fever and no progression, and find yourself transferring to the hospital for a C-section?
I've spoken with as many women who gave birth in a car on the
side of the road or at home long before they ever got the chance to
get to the hospital as I have women who've had unexpected and

unplanned cesarean births. I've spoken with women going post-dates and having to transfer to a hospital setting, women whose blood pressure spiked and they needed to be induced, and women who've gotten a diagnosis of gestational diabetes that changed their whole plan. These stories are not meant to scare you but to share with you the reality that we can plan and plan and plan for birth, but in the end we can't really control the outcome. All we can do is make space for the fact that life happens, and it's up to us to figure out how to handle unexpected changes.

When we make plans, we are doing it with all the information we have in front of us presently. There is no way for us to know what the future holds. Life changes and thus plans change. This is why options, support, and respect are important. No matter how your birth experience unfolds, if your provider continues to share your options with you respectfully and then supports your choices, you can work together when plans change.

I have heard thousands of birth stories, and I've found that very rarely do someone's feelings about their experience have to do with how the baby came out—they almost always have to do with how they were treated during the process. This is why how we talk to and act with women in labor and birth are so important. That experience will stay with us and we will take it into parenthood.

I know because I was that person with a breech baby, and I was also that person with three days of labor and no progression—and those experiences taught me two very valuable lessons. First, that your care provider plays a huge role when plans change. And second, that you should always have a backup plan. These lessons are why I had multiple backup plans with my sixth child. These lessons are why I let go of my midwives at 33 weeks and hired new midwives at 36 weeks. I was no longer willing to compromise on the care I deserved. These lessons are the reason I had co-care with an at-home midwife and an OB for my sixth pregnancy. Having backup plans empowers you to go into labor and birth with the confidence that you are prepared for an alternative situation should the need arise—and that you are prepared to let go of your expectations without blaming yourself because you have trust in and the support of your birth team all the way.

Backup Birth Plans

With my first baby, I transferred from midwifery care to a doctor at 39 weeks because my baby was what's called frank breech—bottom first, with both feet up by the baby's head. It seemed her head was stuck under my ribs. No matter what we did she was not turning, and it seemed vaginal birth was not going to be the best option. I went into the first appointment with this OB, and later the hospital, with a vaginal birth plan, a cesarean birth plan, and a postpartum baby care plan. We discussed each scenario, the options and risks, and what we were all comfortable with. We talked about things like keeping my baby with me instead of having her go to the nursery if we were healthy—which, by the way, had never been done at this hospital for cesarean births, but is now routine practice there. My amazing OB signed off on our birth plans and made sure all our nurses saw them, and he even advocated for us in the OR. It was a good experience because I was supported, listened to, and respected. If I had not had that backup birth plan, this birth might have gone very differently. We didn't think we needed backup birth plans for the next four births, and two of them did go very differently from what we expected. With our sixth baby, we went back to what works: a backup birth plan!

One of the most empowering things we can do for ourselves is to always be open to learning more. When we make backup birth plans, we are doing just that. We are educating ourselves so we aren't blindsided trying to take in and process new information when exhausted. We minimize the possibility of finding ourselves in the position of needing to make decisions without all the information in front of us. We will be able to know what questions to ask to gain the information needed to make informed decisions. When you make backup birth plans, it brings to light questions to ask in your prenatal appointments. It gives us the opportunity to gain more knowledge. It empowers us. That's right, having a backup plan is downright empowering. It's not about letting doubts and fears take over. It's not saying we don't believe in our ability to birth at home or have that VBAC. It's saying, *I will not find myself in a position where options, support, and respect are absent from my birth experience.*

Care Provider

Let me say it again for those who may have not heard me: it is extraordinarily important to hire a provider you trust, so that when they are suggesting a need for interventions you have confidence in them. You do not want to go into your labor having to question your provider's motives. Quite frankly, most providers don't want that either. So, once again, because I can't say it enough, do your best to find a provider who is best for *you*. And remember, if you end up having an on-call doctor or a nurse who is not on board with your birth plan, ask for someone else.

While doulas are not care providers, they can be great at helping when plans change. They can remind you to ask for more information or even time to discuss your options. I believe rushed decisions are the worst decisions. Your doula may even gently ask, "Can they have a few minutes to discuss this?" If the provider says, "Yes, of course, take some time," well, then it's not an emergency. Then you can discuss information with your doula and partner, and you can make an informed decision. If it is an emergency, that is an entirely different situation, and you will need to make space postpartum to process that experience.

Self-Care When Plans Change

Having a backup plan *is* good self-care—it's making space for yourself and your baby in an unpredictable world. You can't prepare for everything, but you can prepare to love and trust yourself, honor your feelings, and give yourself time and space to process. Preparing for plans to change doesn't mean you've got an answer to every possible question or have solutions for every potential situation; it means you've made a commitment to yourself—you've said, *I will only be surrounded by people who treat me with openness, authenticity, and who value my voice. And I will in turn be open and trusting of those people.* You've said, *I acknowledge that I can't control everything, but I can at least not judge or shame myself for my feelings, and I can create space for me as well as my baby in my birth experience.*

When you're thinking about backup plans, don't just think about birth: consider postpartum, too. If birth takes a different turn than planned, this will no doubt affect you and your family's postpartum experience. Things as simple as scheduling help from friends and family with household chores and meals can make all the difference in the world if the new mother is still recuperating from birth plan B because birth plan A fell through.

PARTNER POINT OF VIEW:
Being Prepared

Change is scary. When your partner has planned out the birth and those plans change as the big day approaches, or those plans change during the birth, it can leave you feeling worried and anxious about her health. Everyone around her will be primarily focused on the health of the baby, and you will be, too, but the concern you will feel for your partner's well-being as everything moves at a fever pitch around her can be overwhelming from your vantage point.

This is why a backup plan is invaluable. Not only for your partner, but for you. With our second and third babies, January labored at home with the intent to birth at home. When labor didn't progress in both instances, she transferred to the hospital. One trip resulted in a cesarean, the other in her first VBAC. Babies four and five were home births, but we still didn't have a backup plan for either birth. By baby number six, January wanted all doubts erased from her mind and all scenarios accounted for, so she hired a midwife *and* a doctor. The plan for the majority of the pregnancy was to have another home birth, but we knew that if a hospital transfer was needed, she had already established a relationship with a good doctor that she could trust. The comfort of that decision gave her confidence to focus on her pregnancy, and it gave me peace of mind knowing my wife would be well taken care of no matter the setting.

Sometimes planning for a contingency may feel like you don't have confidence in plan A. Organizing a backup plan might feel like both of you are giving a voice to doubt. Suggesting a backup plan might even come across as unsupportive if the two of you haven't discussed it.

Nothing could be further from the truth. The old adage "It's better to be safe than sorry" comes to mind. It's why we have car insurance although we don't plan on getting into an accident, or life insurance although we don't plan on dying until a ripe old age. A backup plan might seem like you are preparing for the worst, and you're right! If your partner is planning a home birth and the situation calls for a hospital transfer, without a backup plan you will feel like a deer in the headlights and be of little use. If your partner is planning a vaginal birth in the hospital and the situation calls for an emergency cesarean, without a backup plan there will be added stress surrounding the extended hospital stay and weeks of recovery your partner will need.

When your partner is making plans for her birth, make the plans with her. When she makes a backup plan, be there as well. If she doesn't have a backup plan, suggest helping her with one. You have been supportive and involved every step of the way to this point, and you don't want to feel like you're the only one who can't help if an unforeseen circumstance arises during labor.

PART THREE

Taking Back Postpartum

You do not have to be perfect. You just have to be open to growing on the journey.

If there is one section anyone reads in this book, this is the section I want you to read. Because while pregnancy is on average nine months long and while birth is an incredibly important experience in your life, postpartum is the beginning of your parenthood journey. It's the beginning of the rest of your life. You begin your postpartum journey while you're healing from the birth, functioning on a lack of sleep, and all of a sudden you're responsible for a human being! That is scary and big. This is the time where it's hardest to ask for help, yet this part of the journey is where you probably need the most support, grace, and space to grow as a human being. Because the truth is, the first few years of postpartum are going to pull you so far away from who you used to be—and then they're going to put you back together as the person you're supposed to become. It's a magical journey, but it's also one that requires a lot of love and support.

If you are picking up this book past six weeks postpartum, this section is for you. If you are picking up this book one year postpartum, this section is for you. If you are picking up this book ten years postpartum—it's still for you. It's not a week-by-week guide to how your baby is going to be growing. It's a friend to hold your hand and say, "I've been there, too, and your experiences are a variation of normal. Let's push past any pain or shame you're feeling and get you the support you need." I've walked this path many times in many ways, and I want to walk with you now as you navigate your own path. Within these pages you will find a safe space to fall, lean, cry, and just be you.

Chapter 9

Postpartum Without Fear

. . . .

It's okay to say I wanted this and it's hard. It's okay to say I'm grateful, I love my kid(s), and I'm also struggling and need support. That doesn't make you a bad parent. It makes you an honest human.

So much of the conversation surrounding postpartum involves the pushing of expectations as well as products. The constant pressure for baby to sleep through the night and to get your body back is discouraging and frustrating. The honest and messy parts of it—leaking breasts, staying up all night watching your baby breathe, and having a hard time going to the bathroom—are not talked about. Why? There are probably many reasons, but for those of us who have been there, our lack of honest conversation later may be due to the postpartum haze we were in. When we are finally on the other side, we forget many of the day-to-day details. For others it may feel embarrassing to discuss the messy parts of postpartum.

The unfortunate thing is that many of us aren't even having open discussions with our mothers, sisters, aunts, and friends, so we just don't know what to expect. It's the beginning of the "feeling alone" aspect of parenthood. It's not until we whisper over cold—not iced, but cold—coffee that we had a scary thought or that we actually aren't enjoying breastfeeding that we find out we may not be alone after all, because your friend exclaims, "Me too!"

Here's the powerful thing: when we use our voices, we give others permission (even though they shouldn't need it) to use theirs. It's hard to speak up—to say, "I wanted this, but it's hard and I need help"—but once you do, you'll find it's easier than you may think to find support.

There is much solidarity to be found if we start talking openly about our postpartum experiences, but I also think it's true that postpartum has *more* variations of normal than pregnancy and birth. There are so many life factors involved in postpartum life: whether you're going back to work or staying at home, where you live in the world and what season it is when your baby is born (and how often you can get outside in the fresh air!), how your state/country/province/job deals with parental leave/pumping/ breastfeeding, if you're dealing with medical issues or developmental issues, how close you live to your support system, if you have multiples, your emotional and psychological health, and on and on. But I will tell you this: postpartum is usually pretty messy. And that's okay.

The idea of a "fourth trimester"—and the growing numbers of parents I hear embracing that term in the last few years—has brought us further into the conversation about postpartum, but it still doesn't take us far enough. The term "fourth trimester" is useful for expressing that postpartum is indeed a period of time that, like the first, second, and third trimesters of pregnancy, will include growth and development. But it also gives the sense that postpartum lasts twelve weeks, which is better than what people used to say—six weeks!—but still not long enough. If you look up "fourth trimester" online or in most parenting books, you'll likely find a discussion of baby's growth during this time. Little to nothing is said about the transition *you* will go through or are going through.

Where did this idea of mamas needing only six to twelve weeks of recovery come from? Why is nobody talking about the growth and development parents will go through during this time? And why do we all feel so alone on this journey?

Listen, twelve weeks is when you just *start* getting you and baby into a natural rhythm: your baby starts adjusting to being outside the womb, you figure out feeding (one way or another), perhaps you're navigating going back to work, and you're starting to get a handle on baby's sleeping patterns. Maybe you're feeling like, "Okay, I've just started to get my head around this parenting thing...and maybe now I can do laundry while the baby rocks in the swing for a bit."

But then you've got the whole rest of that first year postpartum. And then the whole rest of your life as a parent! The last visit with your care provider is at six weeks after your baby's birth and the so-called fourth trimester "ends" at twelve weeks, but the postpartum adjustment certainly doesn't stop at either milestone. I feel my postpartum recovery time period is eighteen months to two years, which is around the time my babies usually wean from breastfeeding. If you ask Brandon, he doesn't think postpartum will end until the kids move out! You might feel differently. And that's okay. As author Amely Greeven writes, "In Chinese medicine, it's said that when the child turns 3, the mother gets half of her chi back."[10] I kind of love that. The reality is, it takes the time it takes.

We're not giving postpartum equal amounts of space and love that we're giving everything else. We don't honor postpartum in the way we honor pregnancy and birth. If we're going to talk about a fourth trimester, then I want a fifth trimester and a sixth trimester for postpartum as well. Most people don't even see their care provider after six weeks postpartum. Why shouldn't your provider be there for you just as much after as before? We need a radically different conversation about postpartum if we are to truly support and empower moms, parents, and families.

Have you seen those "nine months in" and "nine months out"

photos some people take—you know, where mom is nine months' pregnant in one photo and next to it is an "after" photo of her and baby nine months' postpartum? Let's talk about postpartum like that. Nine months pregnancy and nine months postpartum. And what happens during those latter nine months that we aren't talking about? It's important to give postpartum its own time, because there are just as many questions postpartum as there are throughout pregnancy. There are just as many, if not more, variations of normal during postpartum as there are during pregnancy and birth. To fully support the postpartum parent, we need to honestly and fully give postpartum the space it needs.

The care we receive—and the self-care we practice—in postpartum is just as important as the care we receive during pregnancy and birth. Think about it: we make all these birth plans, we interview providers, we read every birth story we can find, we do all this planning and education for the birth. But here's the thing: birth is an event. It happens and then it's done. Yes, it's important and a lot of processing and healing are needed, but the birth experience is done. Postpartum is *everything* afterward. It's literally the rest of your life. It's parenthood. And what space are we holding, what planning are we doing, what care are we receiving for postpartum? None. Nada. Zilch. It's forgotten—until people find themselves in the thick of it, and then it's like, what happened? What do I do now?

I repeat: there are just as many, if not more, variations of normal in postpartum as there are in pregnancy, labor, and birth. Let's take back postpartum. Let's bring it out from the behind the veil of silence or the chorus of "I'm fine" and "I should be able to do this myself" and speak honestly about our experiences. Let's make space and time for ourselves after birth—just as much as, if not more than, the space and time we gave ourselves, our bodies, and our babies during pregnancy and labor. Let's make it more than cute baby photos and "get my body back" gimmicks. Don't stop advocating for yourself. Advocate for yourself postpartum with as much love and intensity as you would for your baby.

Changing the Conversation

We have to change our ideas about postpartum and the conversation happening around and about it—for ourselves, for other women and families, and for our children. We can't keep going along as if pregnancy and birth were the main event and ignore those delicate, important first months and years postpartum. What we need is to normalize the idea of a settling-in period and hold space for many variations of normal within that concept.

Here's a very common scenario I've experienced myself, along with countless other parents: we get out of the house with our new baby to get some fresh air, or to get away from the toddler who is apparently captain of team no pants and simultaneously trying out for the drama club, and head to our favorite little café or store where we can get some good coffee, hopefully without judgment. Drink in hand, wearing our baby so no one will touch them—or maybe baby was asleep in the car and you didn't want to wake her, so she's in her car seat in a cart or stroller. And you finally take a deep breath. You just want to feel human again for a bit.

Inevitably, someone will approach, and the first thing they ask is, "How old is your baby?" So you answer them with a polite smile. Second question, "How much did they weigh?" This question has made me realize that we are obsessed with weight *from birth*. And then you hear it, the question you've been dreading: "Is your baby sleeping through the night?" At this point you're deciding whether or not to throw your coffee in their face. On the one hand, you haven't had good coffee in weeks so you can't bear to part with it. On the other hand, although well-meaning, this person just asked you a very detrimental question. You're a new parent (even if you already have children) and you're just trying to do your best, and now they've put an expectation on you that your baby should be sleeping through the night. It's happened to me and I know it's happened to thousands of other parents; this can take you on a downward spiral of shame and doubt and you go home feeling worse than you did before you left the house.

My other favorite question is, "Is it a good baby?" To which I have been known to respond, "Oh, this baby? No, I met a really hot demon nine months ago, so this one's half evil."

Look, that baby that they're asking about is eating, sleeping, crying, and pooping whenever he or she damn well pleases. But you are not sleeping, eating, crying, or pooping when you damn please. Your baby is fine. But how are you?

I'm not talking about a small change in the conversation about postpartum; I'm talking about shifting the entire conversation. Because a small but meaningful change, like replacing "Is your baby sleeping through the night?" with "How are you doing? How are you feeling?" wouldn't get to the heart of the problem either. The automatic response for most of us is "I'm fine." Most of us aren't even asking *our own selves* how we're doing. Instead, I imagine a world where people ask, "How's postpartum going?" And then they listen, give solidarity, and offer support when applicable. That has become my go-to question for new mothers, and women are usually utterly shocked when I ask them this. Some tear up. Because, for the most part, *no one has asked them how they are doing with a brand-new human being who is completely dependent on them.*

With one simple, direct question such as "How is postpartum going?" or "What are you struggling with today?" you might save a life. It's that important. Just being able to tell a stranger it's hard and having someone say, "I've been there, I know it's hard," can completely change everything. If you aren't in the space to listen to and validate their answer, that's okay. Smile, pay for their coffee, or just keep walking.

Let me give you a little more perspective. If your husband starts a new job, everyone will naturally ask him, "How's your new job going?" If he responded, "I'm struggling, to be honest. It's all so new and overwhelming," or even, "I'm not sure if I'm a good fit for this new position," they wouldn't say, "Well, you wanted this job, so suck it up!" They would ask why, listen, validate, and give suggestions. Your new job as a parent and your feelings about it deserve the same consideration. With parenthood the feeling is that we wanted this, so we have to suck it up and act like everything is fine. But we've just started a brand-new job (or role) and we never get to say that it's hard, or that we're struggling, or that maybe it's different from what we thought it would be.

So I'm here to tell you that it's okay to walk away from someone who's making you feel like you have to suck it up if what you really need to do is have a good cry. It's okay to say in response to someone's unintentionally hurtful question, "My baby is sleeping fine; I'm not sleeping much at all, thanks." Or, if you're like me, you can tell them your baby is half demon and sip your coffee with a deadpan face.

Sleep When the Baby Sleeps: A Note on Well-Meaning Advice

Parents of new babies get a lot of advice, some solicited, some not. You'll perhaps hear nothing more frequently than the suggestion to sleep when the baby sleeps. This one, I have to say, is really good advice for those who can. If you have a toddler or an older child, that might be impossible. Or maybe you work and your baby is sleeping the day away with Grandma or in day care, thank you very much. Not to mention, some people's babies just won't nap. Our babies are dictators. A lot comes down to their personalities, habits, and rhythms. It's great if you have a really easy baby and they just fit smoothly into your life. When that's not the case, what do you do? How do you take in and process advice like this without feeling judged or inadequate?

Look, if the question is "Should I sleep?" the answer, whenever possible, is YES. With one baby, if you have the time to be at home, DO IT. Sleep when your baby sleeps. It really is okay to let the laundry pile up so you can rest. That knitting project you thought you were going to do on maternity leave? Maybe you will. But choose sleep first. Or advice like this might be an opportunity to reevaluate your expectations once again. What are some alternative things you can do? I'd love to sleep when my baby sleeps, but that's not reality for me—what might that look like in my unique situation? With two or more kids, at least try to rest. Maybe shut off the lights and screens in your office, or find a sunny bench to sit on and close your eyes for five minutes.

Self-Care Without Fear

I'm all for gentle parenting, but can we also practice gentle adulting? The number one thing you can do for yourself is not to forget yourself. In the beautiful chaos that is postpartum, remembering that *you* are at the center of it is vital. It's easy for the baby to be seen as the center of it all, but who is taking care of the baby? You are. You need to process, grow, and heal during this major life transition that is postpartum. You deserve the grace to feel however you feel without judgment or shame, and so does your partner or spouse. You are allowed to be gentle with yourself as you stretch and fumble your way through postpartum. You need to take care of you, too.

We need to start talking about and normalizing the idea of a postpartum plan, just like a birth plan. We need to take it seriously, to think about it, to create space for thinking about it. We make plans for birth even though we don't know how it's going to go—and the same is true for postpartum. We don't know exactly how it's going to go. We even make backup plans for birth because we acknowledge the unpredictability of it! Doesn't the unknown of postpartum need one as well? At the very least let's acknowledge that we might need a backup postpartum plan—that we might need to readjust from time to time. We are getting to know our babies, ourselves, and our lives in this new reality. So we need to do the same: prepare for it the best we can. Create the space for ourselves and all of the numerous variations of normal that will come our way.

Self-care is a journey, just like pregnancy, labor and birth, and parenthood. If we don't think to give ourselves love and care during postpartum, then we're leaving the door wide open for self-judgment and criticism instead. At one of my Birth Without Fear gatherings, a woman standing off to the side, rubbing her baby's back while wearing her in a carrier and swaying side to side the way mothers do, spoke up to ask for advice. She uncomfortably admitted, "I only have one baby, an eleven-month-old, and I'm falling apart. My life has changed so much. And I'm not okay. When will I know I'm okay and ready for my second baby?"

What I said to her then is what I want to share with you now: it's interesting how we immediately start these postpartum conversations with criticism and comparisons—by saying "I *only* have one baby" or "I *just* have two kids." What that tells me is that you're comparing yourself to me or someone else and you're feeling that your feelings are not justified. Hidden within that question is a comparison to someone else who maybe has more children, more perceived struggle and strain than you, and, by contrast, you don't feel you *should be* falling apart. You feel you *should be* managing.

We put so much pressure on ourselves, don't we? So many "shoulds." We see a photo of a mom with four kids all perfectly dressed for church on a Sunday morning or a postpartum body that doesn't look like ours and we feel as if we're failing. Let's drop the "onlys" and "justs" and validate how we feel in our own situations and lives. I said to this struggling mama, "Your zero to one is just as difficult to you right now as my five to six was. It's all relative—and it's all relevant." Sometimes the first thing you have to do is be okay with not being okay. You don't have to be ready to have a second baby until you are ready. There are variations of normal in postpartum. Give yourself permission to feel how you feel.

When it comes to postpartum, we have a lot of unspoken expectations: that we'll get our pre-baby bodies back, that postpartum lasts a short six weeks, that things will go back to normal if we just try hard enough, that we have to and can do it all alone, and on and on. But you know what? All these expectations are based on the lives, selves, parenting, and marriage we had before we had this new child. They're old expectations. They're creating a standard it would be utterly impossible to live up to anymore. We can't practice self-care if we're pushing and straining ourselves to live up to unrealistic expectations. We're setting ourselves up to fail.

So take all those expectations, roll them into a ball, and trash them. They are gone, done, finished. Your life is different now and you need new expectations based on your current day, life, family, and situation. It's okay to reevaluate. Actually, it should be expected to reevaluate! Create new expectations in real time based on how you feel now. You can't fully decide how you're going to feel until that baby is here—until you're in it, no matter how many children you may already have.

And that's the point of postpartum preparing: creating space to love and care for yourself in the unknown. So that if you get there and you're scared, if you don't know how you'll manage, if you feel shame, and if you have mom guilt, you can take care of yourself through this messiness that is postpartum anyway. So that if it's easier than you expected or harder than you expected, you can give yourself love. Just as with birth preparations, it's not a set-in-stone program; it's setting the intention and holding the space for yourself to adjust, process, and heal. It will look different in that first postpartum trimester, second postpartum trimester, and third postpartum trimester—but how you plan to care for yourself is less important than giving yourself the grace to go through this life transition with self-love and nurturance, holding space for what you experience and how you feel.

Are we making space for variations of normal in postpartum? Are we making our bubble of only supportive people who will love and respect us as we learn and grow during this new, beautiful, and chaotic season? Are we accepting that support and help, or automatically saying "I'm fine" when asked? Would you turn away loving and supportive help during birth? No. Then why are you turning away sincere love and support postpartum?

So, give yourself permission, if you must, to accept support and help instead of automatically saying "I'm fine" when asked. Keep or readjust your bubble of only supportive people who will love and respect you as you learn and grow during this new, beautiful, and chaotic season. Your body and life have completely changed; this is when you may need that support most. It's when many of us need it most. In hindsight, we all wish we had asked for and accepted help. The number one thing women tell me is that they wished they had asked for help or accepted the help they were offered. Let us loan you our hindsight and share this wisdom so you don't need to make the same mistake we did. Accept. The. Help.

Okay, but What Is Self-Care?

Most people think of self-care as taking a bath with candles and chocolate and a big glass of wine—and, yes, a quiet, warm, soothing bath is an amazing form of self-care. Baths (if you have a tub, or a long hot shower if not), deep breathing, meditating, and taking a walk are wonderful kinds of self-care you can do in the moment to help you get through your day or week. Sleep is always a beautiful (and ironic) option, too, as are therapy, yoga, reading a book, or whatever gives you some peace and refreshment. Maybe eating a hot, filling meal. Maybe ten minutes to just stare into space, uninterrupted. One woman told me that she and her husband trade Monday nights—she gets "off" at six p.m. one Monday night, and the next Monday night he gets "off" at six p.m. When they're off, they aren't responsible for dinner, bathing the kids, or putting them to sleep, and it doesn't matter that she stays home and he works; they give each other that time. It's not a competition. You're both working hard, both tired, and you're in the trenches together.

If you do these kinds of in-the-moment things, that is good self-care. You are filling your cup as you go. It's what I now refer to as survival mode self-care and it is necessary. I also feel, though, that self-care has a deeper meaning to it. In addition to those moments of peace, sleep, and deep breathing, it's also a philosophy or mind-set—a way of approaching the world and your life. A practice of *choosing yourself first*. Every day.

Now, I know that can trigger *a lot* of frustration and mom guilt. A long list of reasons why you can't or wouldn't practice this may surface. I know because I've heard these reasons from lots of women, and I've given them myself. "I don't have time/money/ energy" or "I don't want to be a bad mom." The list goes on and on. We feel that choosing ourselves first is selfish—that once we have kids we have signed up for a lifetime of choosing our children first. And we put ourselves at the bottom, below everyone else.

It's not even a conscious thing, really. It has been ingrained in us as women and it's such a powerful force, this "good mother equals selfless mother" idea. Sometimes we feel we can't say (to ourselves, let alone to other people) that all this selfless mothering is making us feel unhappy and drained because we think it means we're ungrateful for what we have.

Let me rock your world with a perspective shift. I believe that the opposite is true: *not* doing self-care is selfish. That's right. When you don't take care of yourself, you're being selfish. If you're upset with me saying so, it's because it's true. You're not serving anyone by not serving yourself. If you don't put yourself first, you're going to get tired (even more than normal) and burned out, maybe lose a sense of who you are—and then how can you take care of anyone else from that place? You can, but it won't be how you want, and then that adds more guilt and feelings of never being enough, and the cycle continues. I'm flipping the notion that it's selfish to practice self-care on its head and telling you that it's actually selfish *not* to take care of yourself because not only will you suffer, but so will your kids. Whoever told you that you'll be less of a mom if you take care of yourself—they're lying to you. It might even be you lying to yourself. Do you feel guilty taking care of your family? NO. I bet you wouldn't balk at paying good money on the best diapers for your kid to literally poop in, but you won't spend an extra $30 for a new bra that you desperately need. You're part of your family, too. You deserve that same love and care.

You'll be more grounded if you take care of yourself. You can handle the chaos of raising kids and life in general much better. My kids' needs overwhelm me sometimes. Not because I'm not grateful for my blessings and not because I don't love them, but because I'm human. If I haven't done the things I need to do to take care of myself, then I'm just reacting to it all—I can't handle it. I feel I'm getting caught up in a chaotic storm that is promising to sweep me away into self-destruction. But if I've taken some moments first thing in the morning, before I take care of anyone else, to meditate, repeat a self-loving mantra, or take a shower, then I will find myself in the eye of the storm, where it is calmest. I'm not getting swept up. I can stand in the center of it all and be grounded. And not only for myself, but also as a strong and stable foundation for everything that's going on around me. For my family. That's what self-care is: caring for yourself enough so that you can be grounded in the eye of the storm.

Rather than a laundry list of all the reasons you can't choose yourself first, look for how you can. We all have reasons we can't, so start looking for the reasons you can and the ways you can. It might not be ideal, but what is ideal? Some image on Instagram of someone doing it perfectly? That's not real life.

I'm not saying this is easy. It doesn't come easy to anyone. It doesn't come easy to me. The older I've gotten and the more children I have, the harder and harder it's gotten for me. I work at it. Every. Single. Day. I fight for it. I wake up every morning and fight to choose myself first. I search within myself until I can find my own peace or happiness. It's not given to me; I find it, take it, and hold onto it. Then I do it again the next day.

Self-care will change throughout the three trimesters postpartum—and throughout your life. When you're tired and everything feels new in that first postpartum trimester, it's harder to do it. Your self-care during that time may mean just sitting there and staring for five minutes, a nap while someone holds your baby in the same room or the family room, making sure to eat enough as you figure out feeding your baby too. Maybe in the second postpartum trimester it is leaving your baby with your partner for an hour so you can get out of the house alone, or going out with some friends with your baby if you don't want to or can't leave them with someone you trust. Maybe in the third postpartum trimester it's going for walks or refiguring out yoga or the gym in your new, unique body—or maybe it's giving yourself space not to go back to the gym because you are not ready to face the fact that you may pee a little when deadlifting, or when holding warrior one pose during yoga class, or when the pace kicks into high gear during Zumba.

Later on, it may look like just trying to take ten minutes for yourself before your kids wake up. If they wake up before you, there's this magical, low-maintenance sister wife called Netflix. Put on something for them and give yourself a moment to drink a mug of coffee in peace.

There are so many variations of normal in postpartum that this will look very different for you. The important thing is that you are giving yourself space and permission to choose you, whatever that looks like in whatever moment you're in. It's an ongoing practice. What are you going to do today with all you have available to you? Will you compare yourself to others and get discouraged? Give up? Or will you get creative and try again? You get to choose every single day.

Self-Care When Times Are Tough

When I talk about self-care, I know that some of you, maybe many of you, are in such hard places in your lives right now. I know you may not have a supportive partner or family nearby, or any type of village. I know money may be tight. Help may be minimal or non-existent. Maybe you're a single parent or your partner is deployed overseas. Maybe your baby is in the NICU and needs constant monitoring or surgeries. I understand depression and anxiety can keep you from wanting to do anything, because getting out of bed and going through the motions of the day are challenging enough. Please hear me. Just as a birth without fear will look different to every person, self-care will be different for every person, day to day, season to season.

When I was freshly postpartum with my fifth baby, we were going through hell. Brandon worked as an overnight valet at a hotel in downtown Dallas. He also took care of the few patients he had in our new chiropractic office during the day. Meanwhile, we had five small children in a two-bedroom apartment that we barely scraped together enough money to live in. Many weeks we only had an extra $20 left over to feed all seven of us and get gas for the week. That was a good week. I've been there. It's harder than words can describe. Worrying about rent and food is something no human should have to endure, yet so many of us do.

I was also battling wicked postpartum depression at the time and didn't know it. So, I'd get the kids to bed, kiss my husband goodbye, and sit in front of my computer watching Netflix on a free week (using different emails each week), sipping a cheap glass of box wine or savoring a bowl of ice cream that I used leftover change to buy. And, yes, I felt guilty about it.

I needed sleep, but for my mental well-being I needed alone time more. It's what got me through the days, knowing I'd have that peace where I could pretend everything was okay.

Self-care may need to be something small: a stolen moment, a cheap treat, choosing to get ready in the morning before emails and kids needing you. Maybe for you in this moment, self-care is lowering your expectations of yourself and your baby. Giving you both more grace. Taking a deep breath and pausing.

I've been known to put my kid in the cheap jogging stroller I bought secondhand, strap them in, give them a snack, put in my headphones, and take a walk. It wasn't a baby- or toddler-free moment, but I didn't have to answer their repeated questions, they were safe, and it broke me out of my day, gave me a little fresh air, vitamin D, and some time to be with my own thoughts. Or I'd put them in the car and secure them in their car seats and drive around until they fell asleep for their naps. Then I parked and read a magazine or called a friend. I have a friend who steals five to ten minutes to meditate in a busy park by her daughter's school while waiting to pick her up.

Self-care isn't about money. It's about doing what you need to do to fill your cup, to honor yourself as a human and a woman and to feel grounded. That can be a new pair of leggings, a daily coffee or tea ritual, a bath, a girls' night out, a date night with your partner, a walk while wearing baby and listening to an audiobook or podcast, or simply choosing to pee before you get on social media first thing in the morning or go to pick up the baby.

Your body is literally healing. You birthed a human *and* a whole organ (the placenta) that tore away from the wall of your uterus— and you're thinking you're not good enough because you're not keeping up with the effing laundry. How much sense does that make? Take ten minutes. A whole day or afternoon would be lovely, but that might not be realistic in your situation, so take ten minutes a day to choose yourself first, and have zero guilt about it. I know the no guilt part may take practice, so start practicing!

There's no right or wrong way. The whole point is to do what makes you feel good, connected, and supported. We don't have to wait for everything to be perfect to take care of ourselves. Just start. Find what it can be for you in this season of your life and do it for you. Love yourself enough to fill your cup a little. Be who you needed when you were younger. Take care of yourself the way you'd want your son or daughter to take care of themselves if it were them. You deserve all that and more.

Self-Care and Social Media

Social media can be a wonderful space to connect with people, be supported, get ideas and inspiration, and find solidarity. It can also be a hellscape of pointless debates, constant fighting, judgment, and criticism, and a source of insecurities and unhealthy comparisons. There's one thing we can do, other than getting off it completely, and that is to be more mindful about how we use it.

Approach social media with self-care in mind. Are you taking care of yourself first before scrolling through Instagram in the morning? Have you peed yet? I have all my social media apps in a folder on my phone with the title, "Self-Care First." It's a reminder to me, when I habitually go to click on Instagram in the morning before my feet have hit the floor, to put on my self-care oxygen mask first.

Social media is not helpful nor is it self-care, if it's not being used mindfully. It can be a lifeline to support, especially during the first and second postpartum trimesters when you may feel practically chained to a chair from frequent feedings or you don't have any friends who are parents and understand what you're going through. Yet social media is not the same as a real-life hug from a friend, or the feeling of the warm sun on your face or fresh air in your lungs.

You get to make a bubble when it comes to social media, just as you do with the people in your life. You don't have to be friends with everyone on social media. If you have a cousin who constantly wants to start arguments with you in Facebook comments, it really is okay to unfriend them. You wouldn't be okay with someone always starting fights with everything you say in person, right? So why is that okay online?

If you're following accounts that make you feel bad about the space you're in, unfollow. It's okay. No one's going to implode over it. People survive "unfollowings," I promise. But if reading up on your favorite topic, posting in a support group, or something else online helps you feel connected to the world, then by all means, open up your apps for that feeling. Just don't let it completely replace life connection and support, and be mindful if it turns from something you love to something that is upsetting you.

Be willing to ask yourself, "Is scrolling through this feed lifting me up? Is it causing anxiety and stress? How do I feel when I put my phone down? Restored or drained? Connected or alone? Do I feel held with love and support, or do I feel like a failure?" If the answer to any of those questions is negative, then give yourself the grace to put yourself in more supportive energy instead.

Making Space for Postpartum Self-Care in Your Home

With my sixth baby I found that as much as I knew the importance of preparing for birth, what really excited me was preparing for postpartum. By then I knew—because with baby five I almost fell apart—the importance of the care a mom and her family need in those fragile first few days, weeks, and months.

After my fourth child, Brandon was nearly finished with chiropractic school and could be home a lot. He was able to take the lead with the other three children as we all adjusted and settled in. It was a wonderful time and gave me time to figure out nursing, eat nutritious food to establish my milk supply, heal from birthing a human, and bond with my new baby.

As I mentioned earlier, our situation was much harder after the birth of my fifth child, and it resulted in serious postpartum depression. I remember there were a few days when Brandon was home in between jobs and I just had to escape. I couldn't pretend to be okay for one more moment. I would go for a drive, not far because we didn't have a lot of money for gas, and I would order two tacos for a dollar at a local fast-food chain. Then I would park the car and sob. I ate tacos and sobbed. That should never have to happen! Tacos should be celebrated! But I digress. I would call my grandmother between bites and tears and tell her I just couldn't do it. I'd admit I was not okay, that the kids all needed me constantly, there was never enough time or money, and I didn't know how I was going to get through this. This period of time was when our relationship and love grew stronger. She listened and she opened up and shared her postpartum experiences for the first time ever. Then she would tell me, "January, you're going to finish your tacos, pick yourself up, dust yourself off, and go home to your babies, because you're a mother and that's what we do." With a healthy dose of snot and bloodshot eyes, I'd reply, "Yes, Nanny. I love you. Thank you." And that's exactly what I did, over and over again.

Going through these experiences, I not only knew that I didn't want that to happen again, but I also had a better idea what I could do to help have a better fourth trimester. The space between our fifth and six children was our longest. I needed to heal physically and mentally and even financially. We weren't sure we would have more children. That's okay. There is no magic number of children or years between them. You do you.

Preparing my home to create the space for myself postpartum was one of the best things I did. Here are some ideas I came up with that may help you think of things that will help you! Put together some postpartum bins so that while you're sitting (I liked to sit on a boppy pillow!), feeding your baby, and healing, you'll have some essentials within reach. I made two, one for downstairs and one for upstairs, with things like onesies, diapers, and wipes to change baby. I also added a thermometer in one, pacifiers, blankets, tissues, hair ties, lip balm, nipple butter, baby bottom balm, and any other balm I could find. I added bottled water and snacks once baby arrived. Many moms also like including a nasal aspirator. Add anything else you may need or want along the way.

Something else that is incredibly helpful is having a spot in your most used bathroom for postpartum care. Make a little space for things that will be nice to have every time you use the bathroom. For example, mine contained a peri bottle for rinsing, Earth

Mama Bottom Spray and Bottom Balm (you guys, this stuff is magic, even three years postpartum), and wash and lotions and hair ties. I unexpectedly had a cesarean birth with my sixth—my choice, but not planned. So I added long pads and Earth Mama C-Salve for postpartum incision care.

You may or may not have the urge to clean the whole house and rearrange rooms. I moved furniture around to have my own space in my bedroom. There will be many hours you'll be bonding, soaking in the oxytocin, and figuring out nursing or bottle feeding (all over again if this is your second, third, or seventh baby). Knowing this, you want a comfortable, happy space to do this in. Whether it's your favorite chair in the family room with a side table for your postpartum bin, so you can keep an eye on your other children, or space in your bedroom for those long nights or late mornings, just make it yours. It's doesn't have to be grand, expensive, or new. Simple and comfy with a few things that make you smile works perfectly. A basket of supplies. Also, it doesn't hurt to have Netflix and a good book available, too.

When you give birth, you create the space you want with affirmations, lights, a birth pool if at home, a labor playlist with your favorite tunes, and the people you love who support you. Are you creating a postpartum space with the same thoughtfulness? Spend a little time preparing whatever that looks like for you.

Another thing to put together as you prepare for postpartum is a list of resources. It's hard enough to reach out for help, so having information already gathered can put you at the halfway mark to start out. A list of resources can include your family doctor, OB/GYN, midwife, a naturopath, a chiropractor, different local mom groups, lactation consultant, therapist, yoga studio, and more. Anything you can think of that you would possibly need. Some of them you may be familiar with, and some you may need to research before choosing. This is your backup plan to help you think of different resources and options, just as you do when you're preparing for birth. Options. Support. Respect. In postpartum too.

Partners and Self Care

If you have a partner, and neither of you is getting much sleep—or they're sleeping and you're not—it can be easy to start feeling resentful and frustrated if they take some time for their self-care. But let's not forget dad or partner here. Their whole lives have changed, too. They're going to need help and support through this transition, too. It's not a competition. You're a team.

Our family got really sick when my sixth baby was born. Having just had a cesarean, I needed a lot of support when I got home. But with Brandon struggling with the flu, things started falling apart a little. So I decided to hire a postpartum doula for a few nights—not for me, but for Brandon. It didn't serve us at all for both of us to be sleep-deprived. Sleep deprivation is bad for everyone. A few good nights' sleep and he was able to keep showing up to support me and parent the kids.

While it may seem unfair that your partner is sleeping and you're not, or can go pee whenever they want and you can't because of breastfeeding, the more self-care they practice means the more support they can give you. Remember earlier when I said it was selfish not to practice self-care? The same is true for your partner and the new dynamic both of you are experiencing now that a new little human has entered the equation. If your first reaction to your partner getting a few extra hours of sleep now is a negative one, take a deep breath and remember that it might just mean you can get a few extra hours of uninterrupted sleep later when your partner takes a turn with the baby.

Asking for Help

In hindsight, most moms say that one thing they would do differently is taking help when it's offered. But almost no one takes it at the time. Why? It took me five kids to accept help. Maybe it's a survival instinct—when you have a new baby you want to do it all for them, but you kind of have to keep yourself alive too. There's more to you than needing to eat and go to the bathroom—you're an adult human and you have needs for connection and time to think, adjust, and sleep.

Part of this self-care philosophy is going back to your bubble of support and leaning on the people in it for help. Who can help you follow through on self-care if you feel stuck? Who will totally validate how you feel but won't let you sit in a self-loathing space either? Who will say, "I hear you, let me listen to you vent about that—and let's also go out for mimosas/get some fresh air/see a movie/take a hip-hop dance class. Going to where you find solidarity, support, and relief—that's the most important thing.

Let's try to be specific with each other, because otherwise "I'm fine" and "I'm good" will just keep circulating forever. Make a rule that if somebody comes over, they have to bring a meal or clean something. Make a list of specific things, such as: "I need breastfeeding snacks (be specific)" or "dinner for four" or "someone to do a load of laundry." If someone asks how they can help, you can pull out the list and it may feel less awkward for you. If you are the friend visiting, ask specific questions: "What night can I bring you dinner? Do you have any allergies? Do you want me to leave it at the door and text you, or come in and vacuum before I leave?" If you *are* fine and you are good, then say, "Please just bring me my favorite Starbucks drink and come sit with me so I don't have to leave my house, but I can still feel like I'm spending time with a friend."

Just remember that we are all in the trenches together. The help you need now might be the same help you'll need to provide for a friend later. I have been where you are and I know the exhaustion, self-doubt, and fears you face. I also know you will come out on the other side wiser, more humble, and with a greater sense of compassion and love for others.

PARTNER POINT OF VIEW:
I Don't Babysit. I Parent.

The birth of your first baby, or any baby, can be an exhausting adjustment. Going from "just the two of us" or "three of us" to now being responsible for another human life for the next eighteen years is a gigantic change, but it is doable and a new normal will be found.

It's easy to feel cooped up once a baby is born. You and your partner have to make a lot of adjustments to your schedules and your lives, sleep becomes scarce, and getting out of the house is probably the last thing on anyone's mind. With other children to take care of while January was busy with the baby, getting the kids outside was often the only thing keeping my sanity from slipping away. It still is. I take them to the park and either play with them or stay close by, helping them up and down ladders and slides and back and forth across monkey bars. Sometimes, they find a friend or two and I just back off and keep an eye on things while they play. Once in a while, the parent of their new friend and I make small talk regarding the kids. At some point in these conversations, the other parent (mostly other dads, but some moms, too) inevitably comments, "Looks like you got stuck with babysitting duty." The small talk typically ends very shortly after that, and *always* from my end.

Here's the thing: I don't babysit my kids. And neither do you.

The implication of that comment is that raising children is a woman's job and that as a dad I'm just "helping out my wife." Studies have suggested that active parenting is good for men's health, but also that most men *want* to take an active role in raising their children.[11] It's stereotypes that are keeping us all acting like we're hired, but unpaid, "help" to our wives or partners and not parents in our own right.

If you have children, you have a gift and a responsibility, not an hourly wage. January has often said on social media that children are not a burden. I agree. Do I sometimes feel it would be nice to make an hourly wage watching my kids? Sure. It's easy to be exhausted, overwhelmed, and overly stressed by all the responsibilities on our shoulders. Handling the feeding, diaper-changing, bathing, and bedtime in exchange for an hourly income over a set amount of time one or two days a week? And then the rest of the time I can just get off work and do whatever I want? Sign. Me. Up. That babysitting fantasy usually concludes with a toddler approaching me with outstretched hands, fingertips caked in dried poop, announcing, "I pooped in my butt!" in a sing-song voice.

Being a parent is the biggest investment of time, emotion, and money a human being can experience. Together with our partners, we have made a decision to bring another person into the world and raise them the best way we can, teaching them all the things we feel they will need to know as adolescents, teenagers, and adults. Parenting can bring you a joy you never knew you could experience and a frustration you never knew was possible. The gamut of emotions is wide-ranging and seemingly endless at times.

So, no, I didn't get stuck with babysitting duty. Neither did you. We aren't making any money from this parenting gig. We are parenting. In fact, the return on investment from all the money we will spend or are spending during our children's lives is on par with building an extravagant house on an old nuclear test site. The real investment we make every minute, hour, day, week, month, and year is one of love and dedication that often isn't noticeable at the time. But parenting is all about playing the long game. The ROI for our love and dedication is and will be immeasurable.

I'll take that over a part-time hourly wage any day.

Chapter 10

You Do You, Boo:
Self-Love Without Fear

· ·

*I'm declaring it: if cellulite is normal and cute on babies,
it's normal and cute on me.*

Self-love is about falling in love with yourself. Think about it this way: when you love someone, what do you do for them? You care for them, give them encouragement, forgive them, spend time with them, and want them to be happy. Except this, for once, is not about anyone else. It's about loving *you* on *your* journey: giving yourself grace, finding moments of happy, and getting through the day being your own friend. You're allowed to love yourself. You don't have to withhold that love until you reach some goal. You're allowed to love yourself now, today, even if you're not where you want to be in every aspect of your life.

Self-love is not vain or conceited. If I was standing here saying, "Look at me, I'm better than you"—that's conceited. It's also not about never wanting to change or improve. You want your children or friends to love themselves just as they are. Or even give themselves grace and kindness on their own journey with their mental or physical health. So why not you, too? You're just as worthy.

Self-love is more than how you think an outfit looks on your body. I'm talking about the expectations you put on yourself— as a parent, a woman, a partner, a friend—and everything you're thinking and feeling about yourself. What are the feelings you have regarding your value and self-worth? Can you recognize them? Can you take a good hard look at the expectations you're putting on yourself and the expectations you're picking up from the people around you, and choose to love your imperfect self now, rather than waiting on that ever-elusive perfect?

That's easier said than done, right?

Let me tell you the moment I realized I needed to take self-love seriously. I spoke for the first time at an event in 2013. I encouraged the all-women attendees to find and trust their voices, and to give themselves the same love and support they give their children or their partner or friends. The event went great; it was a wonderful first experience in public speaking. I learned a lot about myself that day, including the realization that connecting with people on that level really energizes me. I felt I had found a true passion. I came home feeling proud of who I was, what I had accomplished, and where I was headed.

Then I saw a photo someone posted on Facebook of me speaking. I took one look at this picture and my first thought was, "Where the eff was this photographer? Did she lie on the floor at my feet to get the lowest and worst angle possible?" All I could see was what looked like five chins on my face. All I saw was fat. I instantly criticized me and the photographer. Then I bawled my eyes out for an hour and a half. I was embarrassed. Inside I felt like this powerful, confident speaker who was lifting up and connecting with other women—but when I saw myself in that photo I felt nothing but ugly and worthless. My feelings about the photo totally undermined the strength and beauty I had been feeling when I spoke and connected with other women in person.

The realization I came to through my tears was that I was loving other women as they were on their own journeys while at the same time hating myself. Ouch.

Since I was going to be doing more public speaking and could not control all the photos, angles, or lighting of every picture taken, I figured I needed to get good with me. I don't mean I went on the newest fad diet, restricted calories, and worked out five hours a day. There was no quick fix here. I couldn't diet myself into loving myself. I wanted to love myself in my skin, no matter how big or small I was, so that I didn't want to hide from photos. So that I didn't want to hide from myself, others, or amazing experiences. I wanted to love *myself* the way I loved others.

I first had to get really clear with myself. I started paying close attention to my internal auto-play dialogue. I found that I was a complete and utter jerk to myself. I said things to myself that I would never allow another human to get away with, and I was doing so on a daily basis! Unfortunately, it's not as simple as realizing this and putting a stop to it with a snap of our fingers. I knew the only way to stop thinking things like "I'll be happy when I lose this much weight" or "If only I could cut off my stomach, I would look good in this outfit" was to replace them with positive compliments. I had to rewire my brain and make a new auto-play in my mind.

Remember in the '80s and early '90s (if you're an '80s kid like me) recording your favorite songs on the radio on a cassette tape? If you messed up or didn't like the song anymore, you could rewind, find the right spot, and record over it? That's what we have to do with our inner cassette tape: rerecord a new tune over the old one.

I found three compliments I felt were somewhat believable, and every time I found myself being a jerk to January, I stopped myself and told her a compliment. Yes, you have to speak to yourself and do so as if you were talking to a friend, because it's time to be your own friend. Same when you take a photo with family or friends. What's the first thing you do? Criticize yourself? Ask for a retake? Do you do that to your daughter or best friend, or do you think they look beautiful even with flaws? What if you started looking at yourself in photos as if you were looking at a friend? Would what you say to her (you) be different?

Doing this was and is a lot of work. It's exhausting some days. It may require therapy, support, and other exercises and help. For me, with each day that I hit stop, rewind, and rerecord, I could feel it start to work. I was forming a new narrative. One morning, after months of this daily work, I woke up and the first thought I had when I looked in the mirror was, "Wow, January, you really are a beautiful woman." This is not conceited or vain. I wasn't thinking I was better than anyone else. I was simply choosing to love January as she was, in her skin, on that day.

Now, years later, when I look at pictures from a past or recent event I don't criticize how I look, because instead I see and *feel* the experience. My mind goes beyond the superficial criticisms and sees the whole picture. I think of the story the woman standing next to me in the picture shared with me. I think about how we connected. I remember holding her baby or rubbing their little feet. If I do think anything critical, like how tired I look, I reflect on how I can take better care of myself next time. So instead of hating my smile or outfit or body, I think things like, "Wow! That was so amazing that she shared with me how Birth Without Fear encouraged her to VBAC or helped her come to peace with wanting and having a healing cesarean birth." How I felt about that original photo of myself speaking—it was such small thinking. I was keeping myself from connecting with people, having more amazing experiences, and remembering these moments with gratitude and love. Just love.

We have a choice every day. I could have woken up this morning and chosen to criticize myself. On days when you're especially tired, after you've been up all night feeding your baby or soothing a toddler (or teen?!), getting a work project in, or traveling, it's very tempting. It's easier to let that old track show through and take over our auto-play in our minds. That's when I have to catch myself and remember I can choose to find the good in me. I can go about my day feeling insecure, frustrated, and criticizing myself, *or* I can go through my day doing my best, giving myself grace, and being kind to myself. Nothing physically changed about me when I started loving myself more; it was all about how I chose to treat me. How are you choosing to treat you today?

Something beautiful happened when I shared my journey to self-love. Other women, of all shapes, colors, sizes, and backgrounds, started speaking up and sharing their self-criticism, struggles, and healing journeys as well. Women who were thin, beautiful to me, who I would have previously thought could never *not* like themselves because of their size, told me about their own struggles with self-acceptance. I was humbled. I realized we all are on our own journeys and self-love is just as unique as our fingerprint—it's not necessarily only about body image or body positivity. For me, personally, self-love had a lot to do with body image. I've struggled with weight my whole life. I saw the world through the eyes of a "fat girl." I judged every woman I saw— her status, level of happiness, and self-worth—based on her size. Why and how could I do that? Because that's what I was doing to myself. For you it may be about your size, your skin, your hair, your expectations of yourself, and any number of other things. It is how you view and talk to yourself. The expectations you have of yourself. The feelings of never being good enough. There are a lot of variations of normal here. Whatever you are struggling with, you can find a way to love yourself, flaws and all, and through body and postpartum changes.

These small moments of self-love are, in fact, big. Not only do they make each day worth living for, this world worth fighting for, but they are healing—for ourselves and future generations. And they are laying the foundation of wisdom, love, and kindness for our children, for we are raising what I call the Self-Love Generation: a whole generation of human beings who don't need external validation to love themselves, who are in tune with their inner voices, and connect with the world with authenticity and kindness as a result.

Body Positivity Postpartum

Think of postpartum like other major life transitions you've experienced. Think of it like puberty: your body changed. Your hormones changed. Your body care routines changed. It was (probably) a little (or very) scary and unfamiliar. Maybe you felt embarrassed and uncomfortable in your own skin—maybe you didn't. But you were changing, and most of it was out of your control: how tall you were going to grow, how that flood of hormones would make you feel, how big your breasts were going to get.

What if you hold space for yourself postpartum the way you wish someone held space for you when you were going through puberty?

Getting your body "beach ready" after baby is fine if that's your jam, but that can't be the standard for everyone. Well, except, I think all bodies are beach ready. Feeling comfortable with your postpartum body enough to feel that way is a normal many women don't get, and then they're comparing themselves to it and it's frustrating and detrimental. Let's stop this nonsense about getting your "pre-baby body" back. You'll never go back to who you were before—we're not supposed to. We've changed. Does a butterfly go back to being a caterpillar? Does a bloom miss being a bud? Nothing in nature resists transformation the way we humans do. Let's embrace change with grace and love, not fight against it with self-loathing and impossible expectations. Can you get back to the weight you were before you had a baby? Sure. It's possible. I'm not saying don't do that if that's what you want to do. I'm saying you have a choice to be kind to yourself whatever the number on the scale, as well as if your hips are different and your clothes don't fit the same even if the scale has you back at that magic number. You have a choice to honor this season of your life, no matter how messy and challenging it might be.

Your body birthed this human *and* a whole new organ that it grew—the placenta—and then your body wanted to feed that baby immediately after, however that unfolded for you. That is a beautiful thing—but it can be scary. You're used to your body looking a certain way most of your life, then over the course of pregnancy it was constantly changing, and the aftermath might have left you wondering what happened. For me it was especially weird to see how my boobs changed. This part of me that I loved and felt very connected to now suddenly no longer felt like mine. I would at times feel very panicked about it, thinking and worrying that my boobs were never going to be the same. Then I decided I just needed to thank my boobs. They served me well when I fed my children, no matter *how* I fed my children. It was my expectations, not my boobs or my body, that were wrong. They were just doing their job and doing it well. It is society's expectations that are wrong. My boobs and my body aren't the same, but they're still beautiful and powerful.

In a culture that wants you to spend a LOT of money trying to keep yourself from aging or changing, I'm here to tell you this: your body is *always* going to change. It has already changed. And that's okay. It may be hard. It may be scary. But all you can really do is see where you land postpartum, and then decide how you're going to feel about it. Think of this as another variation of normal. You may be in a space where the best thing is to accept your body in all its glory, or you may need to get right back in the gym for your mental and physical health, or something in between. What's most important is that your focus is on feeling well, mentally and physically, and taking care of yourself as you navigate all this newness—and not on self-hate and shaming.

Instead of expecting your body to magically be as if you'd never had a baby, practice loving and healing your body. That may mean taking steps so that you're prepared to gently heal from a cesarean birth, such as putting a pad horizontally along your incisions so that you feel protected, or belly binding. For vaginal birth, it may mean making frozen pads with witch hazel and aloe vera for soothing and healing your vagina, perineum, and surrounding areas. It may also mean preparing by picking up comfortable clothing that fits your body now. Thrift stores or clothing sharing can be affordable ways to do this. If you're like me, you'll just wear leggings and comfy tees through it all! Love your body now. Loving yourself to health is not the same as hating yourself to health. If you're on this journey regardless, isn't it better to love and be kind to yourself during it? Don't punish yourself for having a baby and for your body finding a new variation of normal. Your body is going to do it with or without your support, so you might as well support it! With all the changes flying at you during postpartum, this one simple choice might be one of the most important decisions you make in this new season of your life.

I also want you to know that you are not a failure if you don't love your body right now, if you can't seem to accept the parts that you've spent a lifetime believing are flaws. I will be the first to tell you it's not an easy thing to do. But you *can* do it eventually, and I'm proud of you every day that you try.

Let's face it—we are obsessed with weight from birth. You, me, everyone. That's just our society. But your weight and your baby's weight are a variation of normal. Stop comparing yourself to other women and your babies to other babies. You and your babies are unique, beautiful, and doing just fine. Let me tell you something: that woman you're comparing yourself to, the mommy blogger or celebrity or friend who always seems to have the perfect life . . . she's struggling too. Everyone is. She's human. You're human. We are not phone screens. In real life you can't filter out the messy parts with Clarendon or Lo-Fi. Let love be your filter. Choose kindness for yourself first, and then for others too. The older we get, the harder we have to fight to find and choose happiness, or even just an "okay" place most days. In a world of social media celebrities—or socialebrities, as I like to call them—this very real, very imperfect woman right here is letting you know that I have to find that smile every day and choose to love myself, too. And I do. Some days it's easy, some days it's hard and lonely. That is the reality of loving yourself.

When it's your body, the only opinion that matters is your own. Keep doing you unapologetically. Don't even get into a debate when it comes to your body, because, quite simply put, it's not up for debate. You're on your journey and they're on theirs. Sometimes people are meant to be in our lives for a season only. Love yourself enough to set boundaries if needed. Think of it as making space for you to grow and to attract others who are now living at the same vibe as you.

Talk to yourself the way you want your daughters and sons to talk to themselves. Take care of yourself the way you would want them to take care of themselves. If no one told you today, know this: You are loved. You did your best. You are enough. You are beautiful and worthy. You are appreciated. You are not alone. You are strong and unique. You are more amazing than you realize. I speak the truth.

Expectations

There are so many messages and voices out there of judgment and criticism, and so many unspoken expectations about "good" parenting. It can be really easy to get caught up in trying to be a "perfect" parent and hating yourself every time you don't live up to that impossible expectation. Whether it's your cousin telling you that the pacifier that comforts your son is going to ruin his teeth, your mom telling you if you pick up or co-sleep with your baby you will "spoil them," a stranger telling you to cover up if you're breast-feeding in public, a care provider making you feel shame for bottle feeding, or some celebrity seemingly doing everything perfectly— or even an appliance commercial trying to convince you you'd do everything with ease if only you had this new washer and dryer— there are endless ways to feel you're not living up to expectations.

Does it ever feel that if you could just get the house clean, the laundry done, or your kid to smile nice for an Instagram photo, then everything would be okay? Does it ever seem that if you could just get your baby to latch on or get her sleeping through the night, then you would feel better? I know that feeling well. It's good to have goals, but what makes me so sad about that impulse is all the time we waste not loving ourselves and enjoying our lives *now*. We're withholding love and happiness from ourselves when things are difficult, which is when we need it most. There will always be laundry to do. There will always be things to wash or dust or organize. There will always be a cold, a bad dream, or travel plans that disrupt a good sleeping groove. We'll never get things "just right" and be able to keep them that way forever. Life is messy and unpredictable. If you spend your life waiting to love yourself until you meet some expectation, you might well be waiting your whole life. And isn't that a shame?

We're afraid of being judged or others not loving us through our flaws. As women, we are either too much or never enough. Practicing self-love means honoring that we are human, that we have complex emotions and needs, and that our feelings are valid. Postpartum, like all things, is a season in our lives. We can judge and hate ourselves through it, or we can acknowledge that it's a period of transition and change and try every day to love ourselves now. I've found that when I mother *my* way, I mother the best way. We don't have to be anything we're not. We don't have to be carbon copies of each other. We don't have to read every advice column out there telling us how to mother. We only have to be our honest, authentic, imperfect human selves—and let that inner truth be our guidance.

You deserve to be loved at your best, at your worst, and everywhere in between.

I know it's also easy to get frustrated with your children when you have an expectation of how things *should* be. It's as if they can sense you've just finished the wash or straightened up, and they immediately have an explosive poop or open a box of crackers they'll smush all over the floor and call it art. For all the pressure we put on ourselves, we put it on them too: the expectation that they'll sleep through the night, be good at baseball, or love eating their vegetables. But children are never the burden, my friends, and neither are you. The outside world is the burden. Impossible notions like perfect sleep or not crying or fussing are the burden. Impossible notions like having all the wash done or being able to handle it all without help are the burden. Children are hope and love. They are the light. They are a great and beautiful purpose.

Motherhood can feel so lonely—and yet you never get to go to the bathroom alone. In reality, some days all we can do is breathe in, breathe out. Breathe in the good, breathe out the negative. Breathe in the love, breathe out the worry. Let go of the anxiety and stress, even if for just a few moments, and let hope and love be what grows, until it pushes out the darkness. That may be easier said than done. I want to hold your hand during those days, but if I cannot, then can you hold your own hand? Can you pick yourself up with understanding?

Self-Care for Self-Love

Maybe you hear all I'm saying about loving your body and mothering in your own way and a light switch goes on that changes your whole perspective on how you view and talk about yourself. But maybe not. These inner narratives run deep. Depending on our situation and how deep the hurt or thinking goes, more support and help may be needed. Maybe you need therapies or more support in your self-love journey. If you do find you need more help to support your mental and physical self-love practice, that's not only okay but a wonderful thing to do—from joining postpartum mom groups at the local birthing center to seeking out therapy.

It's also important to acknowledge that self-love is a journey, a *practice*. It probably won't happen overnight. If it does, how wonderful! But if some days or moments feel as if you're sliding backward, like your self-talk is as bad if not worse than it's ever been, or if unrealistic expectations have snuck in again and you're feeling like a failure or you're comparing yourself to the Instagram version of some celebrity's life, it's okay. Sometimes we spill milk, to riff off an old saying. And then we just clean it up. If your thoughts slip into old familiar patterns of self-criticism, rather than being mad at yourself, it's okay to say, "Oh, look there are those thoughts again. I'm being so mean to myself." Then tell yourself something loving or do something that feels good, like drinking a cup of hot cocoa with almond milk. Remember that being kind and loving to yourself on the journey is as important—*more* important, even—than whatever goal you're hoping to achieve. Give yourself grace and forgiveness today, right now.

PARTNER POINT OF VIEW:
Helping Our Partners Help Themselves

In today's society, there are many variations of normal in the family dynamic, from the traditional family roles to both parents working, to the mom working and the dad staying at home. No matter the situation, there are challenges both of you will face in adapting to the endless changes that come with a new baby.

But with your partner being the baby's mother, there are some challenges that will be unique to her. You will not have to endure your body trying to regain some semblance of normalcy after nine to ten months of pregnancy. You will not have to deal with the pain of engorged breasts, leaking nipples, or a low milk supply. What you *will* get is more sleep than your partner. You *will* get to leave the house (with more ease) to go to work and interact with other adults. You *will* get out of the house from time to time to run errands or go grocery shopping.

Self-care during postpartum is extremely important. Things like sleep, a healthy diet, and exercise are all important ways to practice your own form of self-care. But your partner needs to practice self-care as well. The problem is that we husbands/partners are really good at taking care of ourselves because we know we need to or we will begin to feel like we are losing our minds. Our wives/partners, not so much. And it's not their fault. With a brand-new baby to take care of, and being the primary caregiver for that baby, it's easy for them to forget about their own needs until things have gotten to be too much.

The person who can remind your wife or partner of her needs is you. Ask her regularly what she needs, and help make sure her needs are met. Begin this conversation during the pregnancy so that when the time comes, if she doesn't know what she needs, you don't have to wait for her to figure it out and tell you, because you already have a really good idea. Some examples might include getting up in the middle of the night and helping with the baby if you have the next day off from work—whether it's bringing the baby to your partner to breastfeed, or bottle feeding the baby yourself so she can get some uninterrupted sleep. Or maybe it's taking the baby for an hour or so each day so your partner can get a shower or a bath, go to the store by herself, or even just hide away in the bedroom to watch an episode of her favorite show. Whatever she needs that day, do what you can to see that she gets it.

By helping your partner practice her own daily self-care, it gives both of you the space to navigate the wild period that is postpartum—together, as a unified and loving team.

Chapter 11

Cracked Nipples, Inverted Nipples, and Bottle Nipples: Feeding Without Fear

....

Breast is normal. Fed is best.

Give yourself permission to love and feed your baby in whatever way is best for you in this season of your life. Bring self-love and self-care into your feeding experience; give love and care to your baby, and to you and your breasts, too, as well as to your mental and emotional health as you figure out feeding. Embrace your baby-feeding journey, however it goes. You and your baby are unique, and you deserve the grace and support to find what's best for the two (or more, if you have multiples!) of you without fear or criticism.

It's time to set aside the formula versus breastfeeding debates and the "mommy wars," and focus on the individual mother and child(ren). We talk about individual care in pregnancy and birth, but forget to do so in postpartum. We get so caught up arguing one way or another. Women on all sides feel defensive and offended. Why are we shaming each other when we should be our own most supportive advocates? We think the world is black and white because that's how it appears on our Facebook feeds, but the reality is we're all living in the gray. Just like birth, feeding experiences are diverse and unique. There are always variations of normal.

Feeding your baby is so raw. It's so innate. There's so much surrounding it because you're not only worried about your own body and health, you're also worried about your baby's health, size, and more. It's intense for a while. Past those first few weeks, feeding your baby is a big part of how we step into motherhood. It's one of the first public expressions of you as a mother. So you're dealing with your own expectations and hopes and the changes in your body, and at the same time you may be hearing criticism and judgment from others about your feeding choices. We can choose to justify ourselves to others and feel guilty and ashamed of our feeding journey, or we can choose to own our choices. I want to help you choose self-love in all things, including how you feed your baby.

I have fed all my babies differently, and I have no apologies or shame about any of those experiences. My oldest child was formula-fed and, ironically, despite what you may hear about formula feeding, is now the only child who rarely gets sick. I pumped breastmilk for eight months and fed it to my second baby via a bottle before switching to a homemade goat's milk formula. It took me until baby number three to breastfeed successfully, and I nursed baby number four until the age of three. Even then, it was not until baby number six that breastfeeding was an immediately flawless experience. I wasn't even necessarily planning to nurse my sixth; but she came out, and to my surprise, latched on perfectly the first time. So that was that. You are unique and your baby is unique—and your body will have its own variations of normal with each child. I know from experience that the best approach to feeding is with a humble heart and a healthy dose of grace and understanding. I own all those choices I made feeding my babies. They were what was best for me and my child at that time.

This is not a "how to breastfeed" chapter. I'm not going to include a latch chart. It's not a "breast is best" chapter, either; nor am I here to shame mamas who breastfeed their toddlers. I'm here to help you practice self-love when you're dealing with leaky breasts and with late-night formula runs to the store. I'm here to give you love when feelings of inadequacy or failure arise and when you're struggling—no matter how, where, or how long you feed your baby.

Practicing self-love with feeding is not an abstract concept, and it's not just about breastfeeding or bottle feeding. It's time to get reacquainted with and fall in love with your breasts. Your breasts are going through some changes, and all this is happening while you're on a feeding schedule that probably feels a little like being hit by a train. Your mama and aunties may never have told you this, but along with the reality that your vagina's probably going to be swollen and bleeding postpartum for weeks as you heal, even if you've had a C-section, your breasts are also going to change. No matter how you feed your baby. Even if you choose to formula feed from the beginning. Some kind of milk supply is going to come in, your veins are going to enlarge, your areolas are going to get darker. If you do breastfeed, you're going to be dealing with leaking, new shapes and sizes, and needing new bras—I've gone through a dozen different sizes in the last few years, I swear. And whether you breastfeed or formula feed, you're going to go through weaning or drying up your supply, and your breasts will change through that too.

These changes are going to bring up emotions. Your breasts are a part of your body that you've identified with all your life—whether you've loved them, hated them, or something in between. Breasts are a big part of our identity as women. I remember feeling that it was amazing that my breasts could make this beautiful, sustaining food for my baby, while at the same time feeling that these things that were mine and meant something to me weren't only mine anymore. Some women love their breasts more pregnant and postpartum than they ever have before. For others it can bring up past insecurities, discomfort, and even trauma. Your breasts are going to change, and you need to give yourself space for how you're feeling about that.

When I ask groups of moms to share something they wish they had known about infant feeding, no matter how different their feeding journeys are, the overwhelming response is, "It is hard." Cracked and swollen nipples are no joke. Sometimes making the decision to breastfeed is difficult if you don't have support or your work or family situation makes it challenging. Making the decision to bottle feed—that can be really hard, too. Not to mention how hard it is to pump, wash, and/or prepare bottles over and over again day and night. If you're breastfeeding, you'll need support. If you're bottle feeding, you'll need support. Similar to pregnancy, birth, and motherhood, feeding is another life experience that can push us to our limits and also allow us to discover so much more about ourselves. It's a journey all its own.

There is no one perfect way for every person, baby, and situation. Yes, breastmilk is a perfect food and our babies are meant to have it. In an ideal world, all mothers would make enough milk, all babies would have the perfect latch, and rainbows would appear when we figure it out. In an ideal world, society would make it easy for women to breastfeed no matter where or how they work, and communities would support nursing without hesitation. In an ideal world, women would feel totally comfortable in their bodies and breasts wouldn't be so taboo. Reality is not always ideal, though. Sometimes it's far from it. What I'm saying is, work hard to give your babies the best nutrition you can, and give yourself grace when it's hard. Mamas need to be healthy not just physically, but also emotionally and mentally. Do what is best for you, your baby, and your family. It's hard, I know, but practice not caring what others say or think—and if you find yourself feeling hurt by what others say or do, take a moment for a deep breath and a little self-care or self-love by changing the recording on that tape. This goes for breastfeeding how and where you please, or if you choose to pump, use donated milk, or use formula.

Don't our breasts deserve the same autonomy—the same options, support, and respect—as our vaginas did in labor? I'd much rather a mom switched to bottle feeding than slip into postpartum psychosis from the expectation that she has to be breastfeeding. The reality is that breastfeeding can hurt. It can be profoundly emotional, overwhelming, and just plain hard to do. It can be impossible to do. And then if you're afraid to get help because everyone's telling you it's natural, well, that's a recipe for disaster. Sure, it's natural, but it's work. A lot of factors go into it. It's worth it if it's worth it to you, and possible for you, in this season of your life. But if it's keeping you from bonding with your baby or feeling whole and healthy, then it's not worth it.

Feeding is time-consuming, no matter if you're pumping, breastfeeding, formula feeding, or a combination of these. Being "touched out"—not wanting to be touched because you've spent all day (and night) being tugged on, hugging, holding, comforting, changing, etc.—is real, and it's a common variation of normal. Having someone who's completely dependent on your attention and your body can be draining. Not to mention that you're getting to know a brand-new little human who is unique. Even if you have other children, feeding can be completely different with different babies, so you're getting to know yourself again as well as this new person. Cluster feeding and teething can be real jerks in the midst of all of this. The best advice I can give you is to listen to your baby and listen to your body. It's okay to ask for help. It's okay to have meltdowns. At the end of the day, no one knows what's best for you and your baby but you.

It's often overlooked in our family and friend discussions that there are hormonal shifts as well as physical changes related to feeding your little one(s). The hormonal shift with your period coming back, your milk coming in, the "letting down" feeling after feeding or pumping, and drying up can be powerfully intense. When you wean your babies, too, there is a huge shift in hormones in your body. I had a huge spike in anxiety and depression when I weaned my kids. Things are going on hormonally. It's real. The changes don't end the moment you birth your baby. That's okay.

That's normal. We have to make space for feeling all of those shifts and changes.

If no one else will, let me hold space for you in these pages. Let me be the voice cheering you on as you breastfeed your twelve-month-old and let me hold your hand as you wash yet another bottle. Let me encourage you to buy yourself a new bra for your boobs to thank them for being so awesome, however your feeding journey unfolds! What matters is that you are mentally and physically healthy, your baby is healthy, and your baby is loved and fed. You are doing your best. You are doing enough.

Breast Is Normal

Breastmilk is the perfect food for your baby. It is, in fact, kind of a miraculous substance, changing in response to exactly what your baby needs. And when you get that good latch and you're producing milk in sync with your baby's appetite, breastfeeding can be a wonderful experience. It takes persistence and confidence and a little magic. If breastfeeding is your goal, I'll be your number-one cheerleader. You are strong and capable. Believe in your breasts and believe in your baby. Believe in you. Millions of women before you have done it, and so can you. You got this.

The realities of breastfeeding are that it can be wonderful, and it can also be miserable—sometimes both in one day. There are a lot of reasons that breastfeeding might be challenging or impossible, such as inverted nipples, low milk supply, tongue-tied babies, and more—not to mention that some women, for their own reasons, simply feel uncomfortable doing it. It may hurt at first and then get better. For all those messages out there that breastfeeding is natural and instinctual, there are as many women who find it to be just plain hard work. Sometimes, as with my sixth baby, it all just flows so well. Sometimes it's an uphill battle. I'm all for the romanticization of breastfeeding, because it's okay to feel like a goddess warrior earth queen with flowers in your hair and rainbows beneath your feet when nursing your little one. Amen to that. But we have to talk about the other aspects of breastfeeding, too: from the painful—cracked, bleeding nipples; to the absurd—pumping in a broom closet at work; to the ridiculous—milk leaking through your shirt out in public because there's a baby crying somewhere. You deserve a lot of support, love, and care to keep you going through the weeks and months—and maybe years—of breastfeeding.

If you live in the United States, there's really no denying that you live in a culture simultaneously obsessed with breasts as sexual objects and uncomfortable with (and sometimes disgusted by) breasts as a source of nourishment for growing babies. If you're breastfeeding, you're likely going to find yourself smack dab in the middle of this. Suddenly everyone you meet is an expert on infant feeding and totally comfortable talking to you about your breasts and your body. You may have people questioning your choice to breastfeed if it's not considered the norm in your family or circle of friends. It can be hard to feel supported through all the ups and downs of breastfeeding if the people around you don't really agree with your choice.

Especially in the United States, women are often judged for breastfeeding in public. And if you breastfeed past twelve (or sometimes six) months, you may also feel harshly criticized for that choice. And you've likely heard horror stories of strangers approaching women to say that breastfeeding is gross, that they should cover up, that they don't want to see that while they're eating. That kind of social dynamic can really undermine your confidence. I dislike the saying "breast is best." That's external validation—who gets to say what's best for you and your baby? But I do think as a culture and as a community of women we need to proudly proclaim that "breast is normal." Enough with all the shaming of breastfeeding women's bodies and choices. There is nothing strange about breastfeeding or breastmilk. There is nothing out of the ordinary about extended breastfeeding or feeding in public. There's also nothing wrong with covering up *if you want to*. We need to normalize breastfeeding and fight the stigmatizing of women's bodies.

Create and protect your bubble for breastfeeding support— those people who'll back you up in public, people you can talk to about whatever struggles you may have, people who wholeheartedly support your choice. But sometimes you fight this fight alone, and for that you're going to need a little fierceness. A good dose of confidence and determination. A tape playing in your head that says you won't be shamed for breastfeeding your baby. That you won't be talked out of it by your negative mother-in-law or friend.

Sometimes the biggest challenge is figuring out the logistics of breastfeeding. If you're going back to work, will you have a space to pump and store at work? Or can someone bring your baby to work so you can nurse there? If you have multiples, how do you tandem nurse? How do you make pumping and nursing work? If you have a premature baby, can you give breastmilk through a feeding tube? How do you make it all work?

I think a lot about the time after the birth of my second baby, when I worked part-time at a local, family-friendly community center for three days. I was able to bring my baby to work, which was great. But when I asked permission to babywear and breastfeed him, it became an issue. The answer was no. Suddenly, they were also telling me I couldn't wear him at all and that I had to put him in a swing for my shift—four hours. Did I mention I only worked there for three days?

That whole situation made me realize that I shouldn't have asked for permission. The moment I asked for permission I was giving my power away and then it became a big deal. If I had just fed him while I was wearing him, no one would have even noticed. Whenever possible, we as women need to stop asking for permission. We're conditioned to feel shame from a young age and trained to feel we need to ask permission just to exist the way we are, and we need to take our power back. We should just do us and then if it becomes a problem, say, "Oh, you didn't want me pumping in this room with this comfortable chair? Sorry." Listen, if men were the breastfeeding ones, would they ask permission to have their wife bring their baby to work during lunch to feed the little one? I doubt it. Women need to embrace more of that vibe.

The way you make it work no matter your situation is you get creative and find solutions that work for you. If you're going back to work while you're breastfeeding, check out your state laws; many states have pro-mom work laws that require workplaces to provide you a clean space to pump that's not a bathroom. Have the expectation that you will meet resistance and go in prepared to fight, but don't give your power away either. You might be in a situation in which you must ask permission, and you need to find other ways to make things work for you.

Breastfeeding doesn't have to be all or nothing. Have that fierceness, but don't forget to have a good time, too. It's a season of your life, after all. You're allowed to enjoy it and to feel safe, happy, and healthy on your feeding journey. Pump and bottle feed if you need a break, or if work is making it difficult for you to bring your baby in. Supplement with formula if you need to for any reason. Sometimes we can become so committed—and I know you may need to in order to push back against a friend, family member, boss, even your own doubts—that we lose sight of self-care and self-love. It's okay not to take it so seriously, too. I think we all internalize that "breast is best" message (I guess that means it was a successful campaign!) so much that we're willing to jeopardize our own health and well-being in order to exclusively breastfeed. It doesn't have to be all selflessness and sacrifice all the time. Breastfeed from a place of self-care and self-love, too. Give yourself the grace and space to enjoy it and to have a little fun.

There are lots of myths about breastfeeding that can undermine your confidence and hurt your mental health. Let me tell you this: pumping doesn't necessarily reflect your milk supply. We are so obsessed with quantifying women's bodies—in pounds and in ounces. If you're pumping and don't feel you're measuring up—or if a care provider makes you feel inadequate—it's okay to refuse that shame. If you do have a low milk supply, it doesn't mean you can't still breastfeed. It may just mean you need to supplement. Supplementing can actually help breastfeeding succeed. And that's okay. It doesn't mean you've failed. Reject any message that tells you your body is inadequate or not good enough. That voice has no place in your head or in your bubble of support. Your body is strong and capable. It is miraculous.

If you do have to pump, here's a helpful tip: they have different-size cups—the part that goes on your boobs—for pumps. It's not your boobs that don't fit the cup. It's the cup that doesn't fit your boobs. Reach out to a lactation consultant or other care provider who can get you a better fit.

You also always hear that breastfeeding helps you lose weight. Again, why are we so obsessed with weight loss? It may be true that breastfeeding will help you lose weight. Some women even feel their uterus shrinking while they breastfeed in those first weeks. Breastfeeding may also make you gain weight because it makes you ravenously hungry. There are variations of normal in breastfeeding; it won't look the same on all bodies or with all babies. There is nothing wrong with you if your experience isn't the same as someone else's or like that of your previous babies.

If at any point you find that breastfeeding is no longer right for you or your baby, then it's not right. It's okay to grieve and feel whatever you need to feel when breastfeeding doesn't work out. It's okay to let go of some of that fierce persistence you had as you fought to nurse, too. Honor yourself for having the awareness and courage to change course so that you can love yourself and your baby better.

Fed Is Best

Everything I said about breastfeeding mamas goes for formula-feeding mamas, too. Your body is strong and capable. You are wise and courageous. You don't need permission from anyone to choose what is best for you—but if you feel you do, then I give it to you. Your journey won't necessarily look the same as that of someone who's breastfeeding, but don't let anyone tell you that by comparison bottle feeding is easy or that you don't need support. It takes the same commitment, persistence, and self-love to bottle feed as it does to breastfeed. We all have struggles and we all need help. You are a goddess warrior earth queen with flowers in your hair and rainbows beneath your feet when bottle feeding your little one, too. No more comparison, no more shame.

The breast is normal, but fed is best. If you formula feed your baby because you choose to for your mental and emotional health or because you are unable to breastfeed for any reason, it doesn't mean you failed. If your milk supply dried up or if your baby didn't latch, that's just another variation of normal. It happens. Sometimes it's not a latch issue or a supply issue, but it just feels straining to have a human so attached to and dependent on you. Your emotional and psychological feelings are as valid as your physical feelings. If your body just says "no thank you," if your economic or family situation made formula feeding preferable—it's okay. Sometimes pumping and/or using formula is a really powerful way to share the challenges of postpartum with your partner or spouse. One of Brandon's favorite memories with our bottle-fed babies is the way he cradled them in his dad holds and fed them. He would cross one ankle over the other knee and make a safe "pocket" to lay our baby's head down on his calf, so that baby would be cradled with a slight incline. He'd feed our baby while I took a shower or made dinner, or just sat on the couch next to him to watch a movie. We all have our paths to walk. Sometimes ensuring a healthy mom and a healthy baby means formula.

Sometimes it means a combination of breastfeeding and formula—or pumping breastmilk and using formula. Give yourself the space and grace to feel your feelings and feed your baby the best way for you.

I once spoke with a college professor who teaches and researches infant feeding. She shared that when she tells people about her courses on breastfeeding—whether it's at a community discussion of the film *Breastmilk* or a casual conversation at the grocery store checkout—women who formula fed their babies express feelings of guilt and anger about their choice. Some of these mamas, she said, had their babies more than twenty years ago, but they're still carrying around that pain. How devastating to hear that the efforts to support breastfeeding have (unintentionally or not) made formula-feeding women feel such shame. This is not good care. This is not good community.

Formula-feeding moms often experience shame or failure because they aren't breastfeeding, a feeling that can evolve into full-blown depression. As I see every year during World Breastfeeding Week (and, honestly, in almost every post or conversation I have about formula feeding), many breastfeeding advocates argue that if new mothers don't breastfeed, they have not tried everything. This is damaging on so many levels.

So you'll need to be just as fierce about creating and protecting your space if you formula feed. Create your bubble of support and kick out anyone who doesn't support you. Refuse to be shamed by care providers, friends, family, or anyone who criticizes your journey.

Care Providers and Support for Feeding

There are lots of resources out there for feeding support—from support communities such as La Leche League (LLL) and Mocha Moms, Inc., to Women, Infants, and Children (WIC) programs, which provide supplemental foods, health care referrals, and nutrition education for low-income pregnant, breastfeeding, and non-breastfeeding postpartum women, and to infants and children up to age five. You can also find a local IBCLC (International Board Certified Lactation Consultant) who can help you figure out everything from latching issues to the best breast pump for you. There is also online support in the form of forums and groups—in addition to Birth Without Fear, there are websites and Facebook pages, such as The Fearless Formula Feeder and Black Women Do Breastfeed.

In combination with your pediatrician, OB, midwives, doula—anyone on your team of care providers—these organizations, programs, and online communities and the people in them can be wonderful sources of emotional support as well as resources for information on things like where to buy or rent a breast pump, local and state laws about pumping or nursing at work or in public, and discussions about brands and cost of formula. Depending on the group or individual, they can also be places you can reach out to any time of day or night with a question or for some love and support.

Treat your IBCLC, your WIC coordinator, and anyone else you reach out to for support the same way you'd treat any care provider. There are wonderful IBCLCs and not-so-wonderful ones. There are fabulous LLL chapters and not-so-fabulous chapters. If a care provider is making you feel shame because of your weight, your milk supply, your decision to supplement, or anything else, then they don't belong on your team. You deserve to be treated with respect and to have your voice matter. Approach any social media support groups or pages with the same self-love you'd bring to social media generally—if it's not a source of support, then it's not a healthy space for you.

Self-Care with Feeding

The number-one thing you can do to practice self-care with feeding is to feed the way that best supports your child's health as well as your own—both physically and mentally. Beyond that, you can practice self-care with things like nipple balm and nipple shields, a comfortable bra that fits your body in this season of your life, and creating a happy space in your home, at work, and wherever you'll likely be feeding so that you can be as comfortable as possible. Sometimes self-care in feeding means asking for help—having someone pick up coffee or food because you're kind of stuck in that comfy chair, or just having someone who will listen as you vent. Sometimes it means having someone else feed your baby, however that looks for you. Give yourself that grace if needed.

Self-care in feeding may look like getting a pump that fits your body or bottles that make cleaning a little easier. It may simply be letting go of any guilt you're having in how you are feeding your baby because you are feeding and caring for and loving your baby, and that is beautiful.

PARTNER POINT OF VIEW:
Is There Anything I Can Even Do?

The short answer is yes.

But there is always more than a short answer when it comes to feeding the baby. First and foremost is that feeding the baby is, without a doubt, one of the most challenging aspects of being a new parent.

That probably has you wondering why I would say it was a challenging aspect of parenthood since I'm a dad and I can't breastfeed. The truth is, neither could January with our first two kids. Maybe your partner can't either. Maybe she has a low milk supply, or the baby can't latch on properly, or her nipples are cracking and bleeding so badly that it's too painful for her to nurse the baby. The inability to get the hang of breastfeeding for whatever reason, in and of itself, can be such a burden for your partner to carry. It is a burden that can severely damage her self-esteem if you are not there to pick her up and reassure her that she is no less a mother if she can't breastfeed. It happens, and it happens to a lot of women.

But we live in a day and age where there are alternatives. Because there *are* alternatives, it's your job to remind your wife or partner of this fact, and assure her that actually feeding the baby is what's important, not so much the "how." Especially if she is anguishing over the "how." Our first child couldn't latch on to the breast properly and it was too emotionally and physically painful for January to breastfeed our second child. Since January had such an abundant supply of breastmilk, she pumped from weeks to months with each child, filling up bottles so that not only could she feed the baby, but I could, too. In both cases, January's emotional struggle over not figuring out breastfeeding was alleviated, and I not only got to support her, but share the feeding responsibility as well.

If your partner can't or doesn't wish to breastfeed, then it's a good thing we live in a time where there is really excellent formula to turn to. It can be a case of trial and error for a few weeks to find out which one your baby can digest the best, but it's worth it to make sure the baby is fed and that your partner's peace of mind is intact. After about two months of January pumping breastmilk for our oldest child (she pumped even longer than that for our second child!), we then turned to formula until our daughter was old enough to move on to solid foods. There can be a stigma in natural parenting communities that formula can't substitute for breastmilk, that it isn't as healthy, etc. This is a burden that can also weigh heavily on your partner, but the key to remember is that the baby *just needs to eat*. And I am here to tell you that our oldest child, a teenager now, has always been our healthiest child.

If your partner, and possibly you, *are* resistant to the idea of turning to formula, you can always look into milk-sharing programs as well as milk banks. Many women have such an overabundance of breastmilk that they choose to pump it and donate it. The milk banks do very thorough background checks to make sure the breastmilk being donated is safe for other mothers to feed to their babies. If this is an option for your family, assist your wife or partner in researching this option.

January nursed the rest of our kids, but it wasn't until our sixth baby that she felt that breastfeeding was an effortless process. It takes a lot of work to breastfeed a baby, and that's *if* your partner and the baby get the hang of it from the get-go. In the beginning, your partner won't get more than two or three hours of sleep at a time (usually). There are other factors that may or may not be a challenge as well, like positioning of the baby, moving the baby over from one breast to the other, achy upper back muscles from hunching over while sitting up to nurse, engorgement, and, as I mentioned before, cracked and/or bleeding nipples.

While you won't have to worry about such difficulties, you will definitely worry about your partner's well-being. You will want her to be okay, both physically and mentally. What you can do is be ready to get her what she needs. If you have to get up in the middle of the night to bring her the baby, then do it. If she needs her sore and achy neck and shoulders rubbed while breastfeeding, then do it. If your partner needs you to make her extra meals or order takeout because breastfeeding is burning up calories like a furnace, then do it. If she is feeling worn-out and less than beautiful and needs you to give her extra assurance that you do still find her attractive, then do it. If she is on the verge of giving up on breastfeeding if you don't hurry over to Walmart and get her nipple shields because her nipples are raw and inflamed and it's eleven o'clock on a weeknight, then do it! Whatever you need to do to make her breastfeeding experience any easier, do it!

Diet is such a huge part of our lives as adults, so it only makes sense that the baby's diet is a huge aspect of parenthood from the moment he/she exits the womb. There is so much more to feeding from a partner's perspective that there just isn't enough room to fit it all right here.

Be ready to assist your partner with feeding the baby, however you can and whenever you can. Just ask what she needs and she'll tell you. And even if you don't ask, she'll still tell you. So just say yes, and do it!

Chapter 12

You Are Not Alone:
Mental Health Without Fear

· ·

I am loving myself more so I can love you more.

I f you feel you aren't enough, if you feel broken, if you feel worthless, if you feel your family would be better off without you, if you feel you're trying everything and you still aren't yourself or okay, I'm here to tell you I love you. I see you. I validate you. I will hold space for you as you process and get the help you deserve. You are not alone. Your journey is normal. Don't give up.

Mental health matters. Society needs to catch the hell up. If you're not okay, that's okay. That's a variation of normal. No more shame. No more silence. I'm writing this for all of you who are not feeling okay but feel you have to appear as if you are. We can be strong people and also have breakdowns. We can be amazing and still feel lost. We can be giving our all and feel it's never enough. We can have happy moments and good days, even when dealing with shit. We can be vulnerable. Because we won't get better until we're honest with ourselves and those who love us.

If you feel angry, hurt, overwhelmed, anxious, or lost, you don't need to pretend otherwise. Your feelings are valid. You don't need to be ashamed of being human. You don't always have to have it together or be positive and strong all the damn time. You can be tender and give yourself grace. You can love your body and your mind. You can be your own best friend. You can heal.

What is the point of all we share when we aren't being honest? My life has been full of trauma and I never ever speak about it. The last two years alone broke me. I have given all I have to give. Now I'm putting my pieces back together and the cracks and imperfections are the experience, humility, and love. They are my strength and beauty. They make me...me. I'm not ashamed of my flaws; I'm embracing them. I have hope and love and will never ever give up. As I heal and love myself, I'll then have more to give once more.

You may struggle as a new mother. It's a variation of normal. You are not alone. It can't be said enough. It is a variation of normal. You are not the only one going through what you are or having the feelings you do. You may feel alone, but you are not alone.

From postpartum depression (PPD) to postpartum psychosis (PPP), from postpartum obsessive compulsive disorder (OCD) to post-traumatic stress disorder (PTSD) caused by birth trauma, there are a range of mental health concerns that can come with pregnancy, birth, and postpartum. Mental health isn't just a question of diagnosable issues, although getting the right diagnosis and the right help are a big part of the work we must do to end the stigma. But you may also be struggling with mental issues that won't reach the level of diagnosis, and that struggle is just as valid. You may feel anxiety, loneliness, depression, or fear of being judged as an incompetent mother or someone to be avoided, even shunned.

It is no longer acceptable to ignore this vitally important topic. Our attitude in the United States has been to keep mental illness hush-hush and to always present yourself with your best foot forward. Many women keep quiet about their struggles. Let me be a support person in your life and a voice in your head letting you know that I've been there. It's hard. It can be such a daunting thing, feeling those feelings, acknowledging the struggle, asking for help, and working on healing. It's a journey toward health and it won't always look like a straight line. I want to hold your hand through it—through your best times and your worst times, because you deserve to be loved and supported through it all.

We must resist the stigma and fight the silences around postpartum and mental health. But it's hard to be vulnerable and share what we're going through. It's hard to push through the expectations society has put on us or that we put on ourselves. It's even harder to share when we are going through it—that is, if we can even recognize it when we're in the midst of it. Sometimes when we are in it, it's nearly impossible to see things clearly. After my fifth child, I experienced anxiety, but I didn't label it as such or talk about it with anyone. We as a society were barely talking about postpartum depression at that time, much less anything else. So I chalked these feelings up to just being nervous that I now had five children to keep safe! "This is probably normal, right?" I thought.

When I became pregnant with my sixth baby, those feelings of panic, the racing thoughts of my children being hurt, and an overall feeling of not being safe intensified. After our baby was born, these feelings didn't go away, but instead persisted. I was certain that something bad was going to happen to my new baby or my youngest son. I'd wake up panicked and hysterical that one of them had died. I felt alone and silly for feeling this way; I worried that no one else would take me seriously either.

Somehow this time around I came to the realization that I needed to talk about it with someone who would listen without judgment. I knew I needed support. About six months postpartum, I decided to text my midwife to get recommendations for professionals who could help me. As I typed a message to her, a huge wave of shame overcame me. I felt completely enveloped in this shame. I started crying. All I could feel was a sense that I wasn't being good enough. And then another thought: "This is ridiculous! I tell thousands of women regularly not to feel shame and get the help they deserve! And here I am feeling ashamed?" It was in that moment that I understood how deeply ingrained it is in us to feel shame.

How even when we think we're completely aware of it and we speak often of overcoming it, those feelings of not being good enough can and will surface. It's a very powerful force, this subconscious belief that we should be able to handle everything on our own, that we have to be good or even perfect in order to be loved.

I can't tell you that on that day I silenced the nagging voice of shame completely. What I did do, though, was hit SEND on that text message anyway. So often we hear people say, "Don't be ashamed" when we're struggling. That message is good—that's part of our collective process toward ending the stigma. But I feel that sometimes that encouragement can make us feel bad if we do feel shame. So I say, if you feel shame for needing help, that's okay, ask for it anyway. You may in fact feel shame no matter how many people or bloggers or Pinterest articles tell you not to. You may feel awful speaking your truth out loud. Get help anyway. I did. You can.

And you know what? My midwife texted back almost immediately with support and suggestions. I talked to my midwife, discussed medications with my OB, saw a homeopath, a chiropractor, and a therapist. I still deal with anxiety, but my husband and I have a better understanding of it and what helps alleviate it, and I remind myself that I deserve to take care of myself. That my family needs me to. And this is why self-care, even in mental health, is never selfish. It's necessary.

Sometimes you just have to feel. We can't always step around the issue but instead have to go right through it. The answer isn't always to avoid or even to get over something, but to allow space for it. It may be messy and scary and hard, but that's okay. You may feel embarrassed or ashamed. That's okay, too. Life is messy and scary and hard. But if we allow ourselves space to move through it (whatever "it" is for you), we can find clarity and beauty, and that makes it worth it. Don't give up.

I'm sorry it's hard. I hate that you feel alone. I'm devastated that the world is failing you. Even still, I believe in you and your power. I admire your strength to be a warrior and survivor. I know what you have inside you and there's so much good. I promise there is joy to come in your future and there are reasons to keep going even if you can't see them. If you must, hold onto my knowledge of that for you. It's through the brokenness that we get to put ourselves back together, with love and strength, the way WE want to be.

Changing the Conversation

In the last five years, as I've been speaking at events, the number of people who will admit they are experiencing anxiety has increased exponentially. More times than not, women are speaking up and getting the help they need, and all that wisdom and experience you gained when you were finding good care providers carry from pregnancy and birth into postpartum. But I also talk to many women and partners who are afraid to speak up because they're afraid they're going to have their children taken away or their worst fears realized. The more we speak up the better it will get. It is scary. Yet we must speak up and fight for the level of support to improve, or things won't change.

We have different families; different partners, husbands, exes; different socioeconomic situations; and different ways of responding to changes in our mental health. Every situation is so different. There's no perfect answer I can give you. Except this: You're not alone, even if you feel alone and even if every care provider you've met so far hasn't treated you with respect. There is someone out there who will. You are not alone.

This is another reason we have to ask more than "How are you doing?" and not be satisfied with "I'm fine." Sometimes the people who look the most put-together on the outside are the ones who are struggling the most on the inside. Bring that woman who seems to have it all together a coffee anyway; she may need support more than you know. So many people are dealing with this stuff. We inherited a huge stigma from our grandparents' generation that you don't talk about this, you keep it in the family, and you keep it hush-hush. We need to throw a hammer at this stigma and shut it down.

Care Providers for Mental Health

If you need to be on medication to be able to get out of bed so that you can take care of yourself, that's okay. There are wonderful family doctors and psychiatrists out there who can help you. Or if you don't want to be on medication, that's also okay! If what you need to help you process your birth experience, your feeding journey, or your postpartum feelings is talk therapy or cognitive behavioral therapy (CBT) with the many kinds of care providers who offer that service—social workers, counselors, spiritual directors, and psychologists—that's okay. If you want to talk to alternative medical practitioners such as acupuncturists, Ayurvedic practitioners, or yoga therapists (yes, that's a thing!), that's okay too. If you want to join a drum circle, an improv group, or a knitting circle, or take a mommy and me class at the YMCA to support your mental health, those are wonderful options as well. You are unique, and your mental health journey will be unique.

There are so many different kinds of care providers who can help support your mental health journey. The hardest thing might be making the phone call to reach out in the first place. Sometimes the biggest obstacle to our mental health is breaking down that feeling of shame and getting the help you deserve. Remember earlier when I talked about making that list of resources before you get to postpartum? Mental health is a big reason why I recommend doing that, so that whatever mental health concerns come your way you'll get the help you need, because it's so hard to ask for the help you need when you're in the thick of it. If you did make a list of care providers who can help, grab it. If you didn't, make one now! Use them. Just start somewhere. Just tell someone on that list.

If it's hard to reach out to get help in the first place, it can be even harder to say to yourself or your mental health care provider that something's not working. It can feel heavy, dark, and so scary. I know. Here's the thing: you deserve the same level of options, support, and respect from your mental health care provider as you do from your midwife, doula, OB, or birth photographer. You deserve care without shame. I remember talking to one woman who shared that the first therapist she saw postpartum told her she was overreacting about her birth experience. Told her that she'd get over it. Told her she just needed to take more walks with her baby. Her baby was healthy, she was healthy, and that's what really mattered. Let me tell you: that is care given with shame. That is care that invalidates your feelings and voice. Next she met with a male therapist, who she thought would never understand her feelings because he had never had a child himself. She was surprised to find that this psychologist not only completely understood, but also held space for her voice and all her feelings. He also gave her the diagnosis that eventually empowered her to heal—that she had PTSD from her birth experience. Sometimes you have to see one, two, or three care providers before you get the right one. Your mental health deserves the same love and care as your vagina and uterus during birth and your breasts on your feeding journey.

So often, as women, we feel shame when we need help. We feel we're supposed to be able to do everything ourselves. I won't tell you not to feel the shame that has been ingrained in you from a young age and reinforced throughout your life, but I will tell you to get the damn care you deserve anyway.

Self-Care for Mental Health

As I sit here in this space, I'm thinking about how I could possibly tell you how to practice self-care for your mental health when I know that you're deep in it, when everything just feels so heavy and all-consuming that self-care is one of the last things on your mind. Of course, everything I've been saying about self-care all along is important for your mental health. It will all help. But what do you do when it all just feels like too much?

Sometimes I am just tired. Not only from the normal mom life, the everyday working mom grind, but bone-deep and mentally exhausted—the kind of tired where you ask yourself, "What am I doing all this for?" We care so much about our spouses or partners, our families, our friends, our communities, and human rights. Then we worry about what we eat, what we look like, our health, our self-love and self-care (many of you laugh at even trying to think of that part).

I was feeling guilty about feeling this way—feeling this *exhausted*—and then I realized that's just more of the same crap. Why am I carrying around all this guilt and shame and fear? Why am I not allowing myself to simply feel how I feel and take care of myself when I need it? And so my self-care message for your mental health is this: you don't have to carry the weight of that guilt or that shame. It's too heavy and it's not really yours to carry anyway. It's some old message passed down to you to make you feel small. It is not your job to carry it.

It's called letting go: letting go of unrealistic expectations, of the worry you put on yourself, of caring if you disappoint people wanting things from you and having to wait a minute. They'll live. It's just an attitude of, "Screw it. I'm gonna eat what I want, watch more Netflix, tell people to just hold on while I sleep more, drink more coffee, and take a five-minute break when I feel like I need it." It's okay to get a sitter for your therapy appointment. That's not selfish, that's good self-care. Remind yourself that your kids just want your presence. That is it. Not anything more, and certainly not what all these articles glorifying a Pinterest-perfect world tell us we need to be.

So be too much of something or not enough of something else without apology. Take a deep breath with me, let go, and do something today—and every day—that makes you happy. Because you matter. We matter. And what the hell is the point of this if we don't feel joy, if we don't enjoy it with the people we love, and if we aren't honest with ourselves and each other? I'm in the trenches with you.

PARTNER POINT OF VIEW:
The New Dad's Mental Health

The truth is this: postpartum mental health can affect partners and spouses just as much as it does the new mother. Birth trauma is very real and probably much more frequent than people in our society realize. Things like birth trauma and postpartum depression are not exclusive to the birthing person. We dads can experience birth trauma, too, but in a very different, very mentally draining way.

I am very involved in my family and find that my life revolves around them no matter what I do. I lie down with our toddler at night and, if I'm home, for naps during the day. I draw for my other kids and play superheroes and tag with them at the park, and I'm constantly talking with our older kids about the realities of life and teaching them various lessons that I have learned the hard way in order to maybe, possibly, guide them along the right path.

With all that said, it should not come as a surprise that I am very involved with the ins and outs of January's pregnancies and births. When she goes through trying times, I go through trying times.

Birth trauma is a very real thing for women. I have watched January move on past the trauma and postpartum depression with very little to no support from the care providers involved in the birth experiences. I was there, but I am not a trained counselor or therapist. There's only so much emotional support I can offer because I've never experienced her birth trauma firsthand.

What about the husbands, partners, and spouses reading this? What happens to them when they see their wife's or partner's plans go up in smoke, or when a care provider or someone else on her birth team mistreats her? What happens when we are there to support our partners through thick and thin, but can't support them in the way that they need because we can't possibly know what it's like to birth a baby?

With postpartum depression being such a taboo topic for women to speak up about, think about how much less it is talked about among men or in regard to dads. I didn't even know paternal postpartum depression was a real thing until the last few years. It explained why I was so miserable and felt my life spiraling downward after the birth of our third baby. All the difficulties we faced from hospital staff and the midwife who repeatedly mistreated January didn't help, I'm sure. But I felt helpless and hopeless. At the time, I chalked it up to having some kind of early midlife crisis.

After a therapist speaking about postpartum depression at one of our own Birth Without Fear conferences in 2013 revealed that men can indeed suffer from it, my severe difficulty after January's third birth finally made sense.

Postpartum depression returned after our sixth baby was born. January's sixth birth experience was especially empowering and wonderful for her—nothing at all like her third birth. January couldn't have been happier. But I certainly could. The difference that time around was that I understood what was happening and took measures to help while also allowing it to also run its course.

You won't be able to anticipate when postpartum depression will show up, and there is no time frame in which to expect it to end. It's not easy to go through, especially when your wife or partner is facing her own challenges during postpartum and needs you. It can leave you feeling like a failure and that something is wrong with you. Simply stated: there isn't anything wrong with you. We live in a fast-paced society that demands a lot from each of us. Throw in a new baby, and it is very easy to feel like you can't keep up with the speed of life and need to pull over on the shoulder of the highway to catch your breath. There is no shame in admitting that. I am admitting that.

Sucking it up isn't always the answer. That's how I was raised, and that might be how you were raised too. But sometimes talking to someone about how you're feeling is all that is needed. Sometimes more help is needed, and that's alright. Sure, you can talk to your wife or partner about how you're feeling. In fact, having that conversation out loud is important. But expecting to get the help you need and deserve from your wife or partner is a pressure they don't need—not while there is a brand-new baby to take care of. Getting help means speaking to someone unbiased, who has the knowledge and resources to help you really and truly get better. I did, and it was one of the best decisions I ever made.

Chapter 13

Hey, I Remember You:
Sex and Intimacy Without Fear

· ·

Are nap dates a thing? Because that's something
I can work with.

I f you are a human being in a relationship, both you and your
partner want to feel wanted, loved, and connected. Bringing a baby home means finding a new normal in all your
relationships—and although it's not often talked about, that most
definitely includes your relationship with your partner, too. So let's
talk about postpartum sex and intimacy.

Birth—vaginal and cesarean—is a physically and often emotionally significant event. Birth's physical toll can take up to eight
weeks or more to fully recover from. It alters your body. Your hormones also shift. In addition to this, postpartum is life-changing.
You're likely struggling to find time to sleep, figuring out the logistics of breastfeeding or bottle feeding, and, in the midst of this, one
or perhaps both parents are returning to work. The very thought
of intimacy can easily fall by the wayside. You may feel "touched
out" with a baby (and maybe older children as well) who needs to
be held, dressed, hugged, bathed, fed, comforted, and more, day and
night. It's common to feel strange or uncomfortable in your body

and to have lots of feelings to process. Make space for yourself to process, heal, and get to know your body—and your partner or spouse's body, too—all over again.

On one level, sex after baby is about the physical: figuring out when your body is healed and ready for sex again and when your desire for sex comes back. These are important. But this isn't just about sex, is it? You're also establishing a new ebb and flow for your everyday life in postpartum. Everyone's in survival mode immediately postpartum—you're keeping baby alive, you're catching sleep whenever you can, and you're trying to figure out a new normal. But real life keeps going: older kids go back to school, one or both of you go back to work, and you have to find your way into your (changed) relationship again. I often hear couples say they find themselves looking up at their partner or spouse one day and feeling like, "Oh, I remember you. Kind of. I don't even know if I like you anymore. I don't know if I like *myself* anymore." So it's not just a question of when you get your libido back. In an ideal world, sex and intimacy postpartum would be a joyful journey back to closeness, with plenty of fireworks and unicorns prancing about. Okay, that might be awkward. In truth, a lot of intimacy postpartum is a sort of awkward searching for who you are right now and who your partner is right now.

People ask me, "January, how do you find time to have sex with six kids?" I answer with, "How can we *not* find the time to have sex when we have to take care of six kids?!" We have to reconnect as a couple. We have to remember that we are both individually human, but also an adult couple who like each other! Let me tell you what we did, and maybe you can find some inspiration for hidden, magical moments in your daily life.

Bedtime can be the hardest time of the day, depending on your children's ages and personalities. After we had our sixth baby, and I was healing from the birth (and we settled into our new normal), I realized we were not being intimate as much as I wanted. A typical evening would be nursing the baby to sleep and settling her in our bed or her bassinet, then moving on to bath and bedtime routines for our next younger three kids. Once the four youngest were all in bed, we spent a little while with our oldest two until it was time to settle down and read with them in their rooms. Finally, Brandon and I could sit down and just breathe. Frazzled, but another day done. High five for us! Then we'd want to unwind with an uninterrupted meal or show or both. Soon into this time the baby would naturally stir and wake for another feeding. If it was before I wanted to sleep, I'd feed her and get her back to sleep. If it was later or if she didn't want to settle easily, I'd just go to bed. No time for sex or intimacy there, right?

Well, one evening as I sat down to breathe with no one needing anything from me, I realized we had a window—an amazing, magical moment in time after getting the older five to bed and before baby would wake up for a late-night feed. That was it! I told Brandon, "Do not sit down, do not eat, do not put on a show, do not pass Go and collect $200. You, me, master bedroom closet NOW!" It was the only private room in the house with a lock on the door. (Don't worry—it's a spacious closet!) We had found time to make love and reconnect as an adult couple.

Eventually, I actually decided to put an air mattress in our closet for these moments we stole away. It would be propped up when not in use and easily laid down when it was that time! Also, the bathroom was put to good use. Instead of parkour, we became masters at naked cardio. It can be hard to find time for sex after baby, and figuring things out again can be awkward or frustrating. But it can also be new, fun, and eventually better than ever!

Sometimes sex and intimacy are easy after baby; sometimes it's laughably difficult to reconnect. These are variations of normal. Maybe you'll fall right back into intimacy and sex without skipping a beat. If so, that's amazingly wonderful. The rest of us are jealous! If that's not your experience, you are not alone. Let's pull the veil of silence away and talk openly about it, so you feel empowered to come back home to your body and your relationship in happy and healthy ways. The point is this: be open to the changes and getting a little creative, communicate how you're feeling, and change your expectations. And have fun when you can!

Communication and Having the Conversation

You can listen to me talk about sex and intimacy all day long, and you can have a conversation with yourself about it, too, but it won't mean anything if you don't talk to your partner about it. You have to have the conversation with your partner or spouse. Out loud. Many times we forget to communicate during this intense survival-mode transition. That makes sense. You're just trying to get through the day (and night). You're working hard to do self-care and to practice self-love. Working on your relationship with your partner or spouse may feel like one thing too many. Yet as a human being, your need for closeness, partnership, and intimacy is part of good self-care. In order to have this closeness from a place of self-love, rather than out of some feeling of duty or insecurity, you need to work at it—and at the very least that means being open to talking about it.

I've found that it's really easy to have the conversation with yourself about how you're feeling about intimacy and sex postpartum, and then assume your partner's responses and how they are feeling. That is a recipe for disaster. It creates misunderstandings based on assumptions. It does not help in creating a new normal or a good ebb and flow.

For the birthing person, perhaps especially if you're breastfeeding, with everything your body is going through and your hormones are going through, it's very easy to feel touched out. It can be challenging to love and be okay with your new body. Sex is very, very intimate, right? It's having someone else all up in your personal space. And you've already got a tiny human all up in there all the time—and that little person needs you to survive, so they tend to get first dibs. Plus it can feel like, "If I don't feel good in my body, why should my partner or spouse get to feel good in my body?"

Ideally, I would love for everyone's partner or spouse to help them get to a place of feeling happy, beautiful, and desired. But in reality everyone is tired and frazzled—and maybe even resentful of the other person's needs or their self-care. So talking is key. You might be surprised to find that your partner is not thinking or feeling the way you think they are. Or you may find the whole exercise to be frustrating, like they aren't hearing you. Maybe try this: instead of focusing on your needs, come at them by asking how *they're* feeling. You're both tired, and you're both making assumptions about how the other one feels. A simple "How are you feeling? What do you need right now?" may set a better the tone for the conversation. Hopefully that will lead to you being asked as well.

Oftentimes, our partners want to fix stuff for us, but they don't know how. Clear communication helps. It's okay to say, "If you can help me not feel touched out by watching the baby while I take a bath alone or so I can go out with my friends, then I will be more likely to want you to touch me after."

There's another side to this coin: we either stay quiet about sex and intimacy or we get too serious about it. But you know what? It's really kind of funny when you think about it. Reconnecting postpartum is probably going to be messy. It might be awkward. It might hurt. It's sort of ridiculous—you're a grown adult acting like a teenager sneaking around. It's like you're getting to know your body and partner's body all over again, like losing your virginity all over again. That can be scary and weird—but you can also decide to embrace the awkwardness and the newness of it all and have fun with it. Have you ever seen those condom commercials that encourage people to make safe sex part of foreplay rather than feeling embarrassed about it? It's like that. You can be afraid of the changes, the newness, and of voicing what you need, or you can make the awkwardness part of the fun. Be creative. And don't be afraid to continually have a discussion about whatever you're feeling with your partner or spouse. Make the newness or the awkwardness part of the conversation and part of the fun.

Variations of Normal in Sex and Intimacy

You may have heard that it takes x number of weeks for your desire for sex and intimacy to come back. I'm not really sure where they come up with these metrics, but I've talked to thousands of women, and let me tell you that there is no set "normal" time for this. What I can say for sure is that there are variations of normal when it comes to desire, libido, and level of comfort with your body postpartum.

The variations of normal when women get their libidos back can be a few days postpartum to twenty months postpartum—or more. That's because a lot goes into your libido. It's not somehow separate from the rest of you. Your mental health, your feeding journey, your hormonal and physical state, you and your partner's work schedule, whether you have older kids—all of this and more figures into your desire for sex and closeness. Remember how I talked about my postpartum time being about eighteen months to two years (not six weeks), which was usually around the time when I weaned my babies? Well, sex is related to that. There's nothing wrong with you if it takes no time at all, or if it takes a while. It's just a part of your season right now. You aren't alone if your libido or your chemistry is misfiring after birth. All you can do is make space for yourself to heal, process, and create a new ebb and flow with your partner. You can't fit yourself into some standard time frame. It's much better to listen to your body, trust your instincts, and be gentle and open with yourself and your partner.

Postpartum sex might be awkward, scary, nonexistent, fun, exciting, new, the same as before, and/or even better than before. There is no "one feeling" you're only allowed to have. It can be painful and awkward for a while until you get your hormones leveled out again, and then suddenly wonderful. Also, just because you're ready doesn't mean it will feel good right away. And that's okay. Once your body is healed and you feel ready to have sex again for the first time since giving birth, the experience can be weird, even painful. It can prove to be an unenjoyable experience not only for you, but for your partner too. The orgasms may not be abundant, and it may feel that you're doing it just for the sake of doing it. You don't have to get stuck in this space; it's just part of a normal journey. Let me validate the awkwardness of postpartum sex for you. There's nothing wrong with you.

It may or may not be the same after every time you have a baby, because every baby—and birth experience—is unique. It might be completely different. You won't know if it's going to come right back or if it's going to take therapy for it to come back until you're in it. You won't know if it's going to be fabulous or awkward or even both until you're in it.

I'm sure my mama never told me this, but let me be the person to remind you that not everything is vaginal sex—if that doesn't feel comfortable right now, that's not the only way to be intimate, right?

Expectations

Like with all things in postpartum (and life!), it's so powerful to examine our expectations. There's nothing wrong with going through a period of reconnecting with your partner, especially after such a major life change—it's our expectations that give us the false belief that everything should be the same as it was before (or sometimes we even think things should magically be better). It's a time of transition. We can embrace the unknown and flow with it or we can set up unrealistic expectations that inevitably leave us bitter and disappointed.

Sometimes unrealistic expectations come from our partner or

spouse; I've heard from women that they often feel they have to be having sex again to please their partners. That's not okay. You are going through bodily changes, hormonal changes, changes in your breasts, and more, but it's also your job to please them even if you don't feel okay in your own body? When is it going to turn around to where our husbands are trying to please us? When are we going to get rid of this shame and stigma that make women feel they can't ask for what they want or what feels good to them? If you're exhausted, touched out, and feeling pressure that you need to please your husband, then that vibe is altogether wrong. Sex and intimacy shouldn't be a chore or to placate someone. We want to reconnect postpartum, and that means we're all on the same team. Sometimes it's us assuming they feel that way when they don't, so again, have the conversation with them.

I remember a few weeks after the birth of my third baby, Brandon complained to me that we weren't being intimate as much as he'd like. By complaining, I mean downright rude. When he said to me, "I can count the number of times we've had sex on one hand!" I looked him right in the eye and said, "I can count the number of times you've been intimate toward me on one hand as well! Have you come to me with any kind of intimacy other than to complain you're not getting sex from me since our baby was born?" He looked at me like, "I have completely lost this argument." Yep. When we talk about this today, he shakes his head like, "What was I thinking?" Hindsight gives us the perspective that we were in a season and a lot of growth was happening. We get so stuck on stuff in the moment we are going through it, especially when we're tired, and then we feel that our needs aren't being met. But we forget that this is not a competition. It's not only about you or about me or about sex. It's about being close and connecting, growing together instead of apart, and being a couple and partners.

It's hard when everyone needs something from you and it doesn't feel like anyone is offering you anything in return. That makes sense for babies, but not for relationships. Approach sex and intimacy with a whole lot of self-care and self-love. You can't pour from an empty cup. You can't always give and give and never feel taken care of in return. So make that a priority. Make your expectations about reconnecting and communicating and not about simply having your needs met or about things going back to the way they were before.

When you hear about reconnecting postpartum, the thing you hear about most is date nights. The idea of date nights is great, but they can set up an unrealistic expectation, especially in the beginning. Sometimes it's hard to go out on dates, especially if the baby needs your breasts or your body, or if it's difficult to find the money to hire a sitter or to find someone you feel comfortable leaving your baby (and other kids) with. Sometimes it's just not ideal or even desirable to think about putting on a real bra and leaving the house.

It's hard to get that time to yourself. You have to find what works for you in your situation. Throw those former expectations out the window and create new ones. Maybe it's watching *Game of Thrones* with movie popcorn and M&Ms while the baby is chill. Yeah, you might have to pause your show three times to change a diaper, but your whole life isn't broken and over because you have to pause a show or come up with new ways to enjoy your partner's company.

Self-Care for Sex and Intimacy

I've taken hundreds of flights in the last few years, and at the beginning of *every* flight you get that same little lesson: make sure you put on your own mask first. And self-care is no different. You're not going to be able to give as much love and care to your relationship with your partner or spouse if you're touched out or bone-deep exhausted. If you are not caring for yourself and filling your own cup, you won't have much to give to your partner or spouse. If you're not taking care of yourself, the last thing you want to do is get naked and have someone touch you. It can cause resentment and frustration, hinder communication, and just get you into an ebb and flow you don't want.

I know it's easier said than done to take care of yourself. Find small ways. You've got to practice self-care to want to practice relationship care. You're half of that relationship—you have to take care of yourself, and your partner has to take care of themselves, and *then* you can take care of each other.

Sex and intimacy can be forms of self-care, too. Being touched, having an orgasm, cuddling, kissing—all these things get that oxytocin flowing. Sex and intimacy can be mentally and physically healing parts of your life. This may not be true for everyone, and may not be the case in every season of your life, but it can be. So put intimacy in your self-care toolbox, too.

Care Providers for Sex and Intimacy

We have to fight stigmas when it comes to women's sexual health. Look, you can Pinterest every postpartum ab workout in the world, but if your body isn't healing well after birth, then you deserve a good care provider to help you through this. Some women have pelvic floor issues after pregnancy and birth; some deal with diastasis recti, or abdominal muscle separation. Doing Kegels isn't going to fix these issues. They can affect your sexual pleasure, your desire, your comfortableness with your body, and more.

After six weeks, ask your midwife or OB how your stitches are healing and/or how your vulva looks. You had a baby and then you're afraid to ask your care provider how your vaginal wall is doing? Go on and ask how it looks, share how it feels, have a full conversation about your body. If it's not repairing on its own the way you want it to, you deserve to go to a professional to help you with that. Talk with your midwife or OB. See a physical therapist if you're having pelvic floor issues. Some women need a little more reconstructive health to repair their pelvic floor so they're not constantly peeing or so they're not having pain during sex. These are variations of normal—help is out there in many forms and there is no shame in seeking it.

Sometimes you need someone to help you with your hormone balance postpartum. There are wonderful practitioners of alternative medicine, nutritionists, and homeopaths who can help you balance your hormones so that you sleep better, have more energy and clarity, and feel more at ease as your hormones and body shift and change postpartum.

Your libido and feelings about your body can be affected by your mental health, too. If you have trauma or are struggling emotionally or psychologically, it's okay to seek help. Whatever you need to do to support your mental health so that you can enjoy intimacy again, do it. In addition to your individual mental health journey, why not explore things like couples therapy or a couples detox that you can do together as well?

PARTNER POINT OF VIEW:
The First Time All Over Again

Remember the first time you ever had sex? Remember how awkward it was? You knew Tab A went into Slot B, but the combination of butterflies and giddiness might have made things seem a little more complicated than they really were. Guess what? The first time you and your wife/partner have sex again after the baby's birth is like your first time all over again. But why?

First, your wife or partner has to heal. Healing takes time. She just gave birth to a little human being who was much wider than her vaginal canal. Even if it was a smooth birth, there was still some level of tearing on the inside that needed time to heal. If it wasn't a smooth birth, then the tearing might have been more serious and will take longer to heal. If she had a C-section, remember that it was major surgery—even if the baby didn't enter the world through the birth canal, your partner's abdominal wall will need some time to heal before you can lay your gut on top of hers during sex. Not to mention the postpartum bleeding she will have vaginally, like a period. And healing time may vary. Some women heal quickly, others not so much. It's not anything you have a say in, so you just need to wait until she tells you that she is ready. It could be weeks to months to many months, so don't bank on any one time frame you may have heard or read about.

Second, it depends on how postpartum is going for your wife or partner. As you have read throughout this book, having a baby is a huge, gigantic, enormous life change that can take some time to get used to. Sure, it might be hard to see the baby getting more out of your wife's boobs than you are, but I can assure you the baby won't always breastfeed and that you will truly regain the joy you get from her body not too far in the distant future. Just be patient, because your partner's sleep deprivation while the baby is small and needs to be fed every few hours can take its toll. If the baby is fussy or colicky while awake, that can be mentally taxing for an already exhausted mom as well. Maybe postpartum depression has become a reality for your partner and she needs major support just to get out of bed every day.

By this point, you know that you can best support your spouse or partner by offering to take the baby for a little while so she can take a bath or go out for some alone time, rubbing her neck and shoulders of your own volition, making or ordering dinner so neither of you has to worry about it, and/or simply giving her a hug and a kiss and telling her she's beautiful. There's a good chance she's feeling over-touched, worn-out, and *not* beautiful, so any of the aforementioned examples might just be what she needs in the moment.

The third reason why sex is awkward after a baby is because you are both out of practice. Because of your partner's healing and the challenges postpartum can bring, the flirting and foreplay might not be firing on all cylinders the way you remember either. Again, remember your first time having sex. It probably wasn't as good as the sex you had to make this baby who has now interrupted your sex life. As January says, you are both finding your new normal, and that applies to the bedroom as much as any other aspect of parenthood, postpartum, and your marriage. Just enjoy the fact that you and your partner can work out the kinks while naked. Don't worry—eventually the kinks will become kinky again.

January and I laugh about how we've had seven first times. I can assure you that sex eventually returns to normal after each child and gets even better than before.

Until the next baby shows up and you're back to waiting in line for your partner's boobs.

Conclusion: The Self-Love Generation

....

Nourish your body; detox your life.

The Birth Without Fear philosophy is not just about having babies and raising kids, or about mental health and reconnecting with your partner postpartum; it's really a whole movement made up of all of us taking back our lives from the fear-based messages that have defined us for too long. We women especially have been conditioned to feel ashamed of our bodies and our feelings, so much so that we often have a subconscious belief that we have to listen to authority, and that we don't deserve to be listened to. The heart of Birth Without Fear is the belief that our bodies and our feelings are valid; that we don't have to ignore our fear, but nor do we have to be imprisoned by it. At any time during the journey of pregnancy, birth, parenthood, and life itself, we have the opportunity to choose nourishment, trust our intuition, do our best, and then let the f*ck go.

We as parents often have expectations that everything we do must be organic, child-led, attachment parenting–perfect, and bra-free, all while looking our best and never not being okay. That is a lie. It's unrealistic, at least for every day! What happens when we don't meet this expectation of greatness? We feel like failures, beat ourselves up, get frustrated, and more. That serves no one. It tears you down and takes you away from self-love. It gives your child or children a more frustrated, anxious, or depressed mom. What's the point?

Listen to me: Maybe all you do today is sit on your couch at

213

home (whether that be a huge house, an apartment, an RV, or the basement of your in-laws' house, it's a home), and no one's in pants (which you can blame Daniel the Tiger for), and you're just feeding the baby, and your toddler will only eat Frosted Flakes that are littering the floor, making a sugary, snowy wonderland while you all watch *Sesame Street* again. Guess what? You have a home, their bellies are full, Frosted Flakes are vitamin-fortified, and they are learning about the letter Q and the number 7! You are doing AMAZING! They are loved and safe. Everything else you do for them or accomplish is icing on the rainbow cake.

We are the ones putting these perfect-mommy expectations on ourselves. Our children aren't. They want *us*. That's it. We are good enough for them as we are. Let's be good enough for ourselves. Let's love us the way they love us. Let us be the mother we needed when we were younger. For them and for us. Love yourself the way you want your children to love themselves when they are sitting on the couch in a similar fashion one day . . . tired, leaky breasts, no pants, and questioning everything. You would want to wrap your loving arms around them and tell them it's okay, and you love them, and they are doing enough because they are loving their babies. Do that for yourself.

I have a secret to share. Some days I do not feel that I am enough. That I am trying to fit a square peg into a round hole. That I'll never catch up. That I'm not doing enough. That I am simply *not enough*. We all go through it. If you're feeling inadequate today, I want you to know that you are needed, you are doing all you can, and that is enough, because it has to be. If no one else has told you today, let me be the one to tell you: I love you. And no matter what, you are going to be fine and it will all work out.

Let's be the ones who prioritize self-love and self-care, so that we're passing down to the next generation that same unconditional love and care, rather than our feelings of inadequacy. Let's be the ones who say yes, advances in medical knowledge are great, but that knowledge doesn't get to take precedence over our autonomy and voices. Let's be the ones who won't wait to love ourselves only when we reach size *x*, *y*, or *z*, because life's too short to spend another minute putting our self-love on hold. Let's be the ones who say that the people in our lives—including ourselves—aren't a distraction from our to-do list: they are our priority. We don't have to have all the answers or figure everything out now; we just have to give ourselves permission to keep showing up for ourselves and each other in whatever perfectly imperfect ways we can.

Birth Without Fear began as a simple passion to let women know they have choices in childbirth. It then evolved to become a source of inspiration and support to women and their families through their experiences with trying to conceive, pregnancy, birth, and postpartum. Now I'm passing the torch. It's not just my passion and my voice anymore; it's all of ours. I've put everything I've ever wanted to say to women and families on their pregnancy, birth, and postpartum journeys down on paper, and I've filtered it with nothing but love. I do this not only to give you information and empower you, but also to hand it over to you so that we become a collection of voices coming together to work for women, our families, and the next generation. Now it's your turn—take my experiences and knowledge, and expand upon them. Make my dream of a birth without fear better and bigger. Celebrate our shared vision and all the variations of normal that make us unique. Expect and give care without shame. Demand options, support, and respect in all things. Filter everything with love. It's the only filter you'll ever need.

Birth Without Fear Harmony Circle Guide

Somewhere along the way, pregnancy and childbirth have become conditions to be treated rather than journeys of love and connection with ourselves, our families, and our communities. So many of us—whether we have a vaginal or cesarean birth—feel *acted upon* by care providers during labor, our voices drowned out by one medical expert after another as shifts change, and our wishes unknowingly ignored by silent nurses staring at computer screens instead of into our eyes. It's not that most medical professionals are unkind or uncaring, but that the medical model of birth, and the medical system in general, isn't quite working. Even doctors will tell you they have a schedule and protocol to follow and variations of normal don't often get factored in, or that insurance companies are pressuring them to take on more patients, effectively doing away with their ability to make personal relationships the heart of their practice.

We as a culture don't understand pregnancy and birth very well, either. Just think about pop culture: in movies and television, birth is regarded as an immensely frightful and painful experience, thought of as an experience to be avoided at all costs. You see it again and again: the screaming wife, the fearful, trying-to-be-supportive (but mostly freaked out) dad or partner, the surprisingly quick and easy laboring, despite the screaming and pleading to be "knocked out." The paradigm of pregnancy, birth, and postpartum in our society is based in fear.

About 9 percent of women suffer with PTSD associated with birth, and anywhere from 11 to 20 percent of women struggle with postpartum depression, but those numbers don't tell the whole story: women given due dates they know aren't right by providers who won't listen to their body knowledge, women who fire their doctors halfway through labor, women told by friends that a cesarean isn't a "real birth," and on and on.

After birth, variations of normal are no more acknowledged than during it. There is a void of information available for new mothers and their partners as the often unexpected challenges of postpartum set in. Discussions of depression, anxiety, and even anger are virtually nonexistent and treated as taboo. Postpartum also adds another layer of uncertainty and choices that too frequently undermine women's confidence and sense of self: Breastfeeding or bottle? How much screen time? Work or stay at home? You may also be dealing with learning to love your breasts (again), working through that awkward reconnecting phase with your spouse or partner, or getting help for mental health struggles.

There are so many ways our birthing and parenting experiences get co-opted: by the medical community, talking head "experts," and even friends and family; or we find that our stories get told through centimeters dilated, fetal heart rate monitors, and percentages on child development charts at the expense of our options and our authentic voices.

We trust and hope we will be *acted with*, that we and our partners will be equal members of a collaborative birth team and supportive community. We take classes and read books, we write birth plans, we have dreams and visions for this momentous experience in our lives—and then, too often, without any preparation or explanation at all, those dreams, and our body knowledge, take a back seat, with no one even bothering to ask, "*How do you feel?*" As long as the newborn baby is safe, according to modern medicine and well-meaning friends and family, the "treatment" was a success.

How can we embrace the wonderful medical capabilities available to us without losing the interpersonal, the variations, and the human element? And what of the physical and emotional health of the mother? How can she learn to trust again, claim her voice, and come home to her body and her identity as a parent?

I have traveled extensively hosting Birth Without Fear events, and everywhere I go I hear the same thing, even when the specifics vary widely: women having episiotomies done without their knowledge and against their express wishes; women being bullied into another C-section when they're trying for a VBAC; women with no options when their baby presented in a breech position; and even women who had the birth experience of their dreams but find themselves struggling with postpartum depression and anxiety without the support of their friends, who tell them they should be grateful and stop complaining. And yet here we all are, carrying around these painful experiences, thinking we're alone, wondering if we're good enough, encouraged to put on a happy face. We have our babies. so what reason do we have to be sad?

"I couldn't do this without you," these moms tell me. "Without you I'd still be struggling in isolation, going through the motions, trying to make my life, my hair, and my body look as good as other moms' Instagram posts do. I would have never even tried a VBAC or had peace with a healing cesarean birth that was my choice, and I owned that because you showed me I could." I'll take that love and those compliments—I love meeting you and supporting community and solidarity! It truly is my calling. The truth is, though, that you *can* do it without me! All throughout this book, I have been encouraging you and your partners to trust your own voices, to get in touch with what you need, and to believe in yourselves. Now I want to help you use this book to gather together, so that the end of the book doesn't mean the end of my support for you.

Sometimes the hardest thing to do is reach out and ask for what you need. With so many different experiences out there, many women are afraid to share their pregnancy, birth, and parenting choices with others for fear of being judged. If you have access to a good support system—whether it's family, a mother's group, a kickboxing group, or whatever—that's wonderful! But many of us feel isolated and lonely as parents. The mother's group you'd love to attend meets when you're at work, or you can't get a sitter for a regular exercise class, or your family is miles away. You may have lingering hurt from past friendships that did not end well, or have a lot of anxiety opening yourself up to new situations and people. If you feel that way, I want to empower you to create your own support group, or what I call a *harmony circle*. A harmony circle is a nonjudgmental space. It's a space for storytelling and healing, for venting and having someone to pick you up and help you keep going.

Here are some suggestions for creating your own harmony circle:

1. *Put out the call:* Reach out to other women in your community, whether it's in the weekly play group you attend, a new mama Facebook group you belong to, or a postpartum yoga class. Getting to know other women in your community and learning that they might be going through similar struggles or have been through similar struggles can mean everything in those times when you feel most alone.

2. *Create the space:* What better way to gather around with other moms in a show of solidarity and support than in a coffee shop? If the weather is nice, gather together at a park. Or hold the harmony circle in your home or a yoga studio with coffee or tea and treats to follow! Creating the space also means knowing this circle is safe. It is for support, solidarity, healing, and validation. It's a way to come together, even through your differences, because you are in the trenches together. You don't have to do everything the same way as other mothers to support and love each other. In fact, sometimes it's our differences that we can learn from and that humble us to be more understanding. The energy of the space stems largely from who is facilitating and leading it, so be very intentional about it.

3. *Facilitate sharing and discussion:* I always tell attendees at all Birth Without Fear events that the first ninety seconds are the most awkward. Even if the group you have brought together knows each other, leaving yourself vulnerable can be especially difficult. "Will I be judged?" and "Will they stop speaking to me?" are valid concerns. But chances are that if you have approached these other women to participate in a harmony circle specifically with your group in mind, they are also feeling their own vulnerability. "Going first" takes

a lot of courage, but you already know you're courageous because you organized this harmony circle.

4. *Binding together*: At every Birth Without Fear event, we place a bowl of beads—preferably glass, but any will do—and colorful hemp twine in the center of each table prior to the harmony circles. As we near the end of our time, I ask one person to wrap it around one of their wrists twice, then the next person does the same, and the next—until everyone in the circle is connected by this string. Then we "cut the cord." I assure everyone it's delayed cord clamping, so no worries! After the laughter at my bad joke subsides, I instruct all the women to gather beads for the important moments in their lives, thread the string through each bead, and tie it off around their wrist as a bracelet to remind them of the solidarity and support they were a part of. Beads and string are inexpensive and easy to find at any craft store near you. It's a way to remind us that we are all connected by invisible strings of solidarity and love. It's powerful to have shared and remember your shared space with strong, amazing women who "just get it." You are not alone.

5. *Stay Connected*: If all the women in your harmony circle know each other, make a point as a group to gather together more often to support one another. If you don't know some of the other women in your harmony circle group, exchange phone numbers and email addresses. At one Birth Without Fear event a few years ago, several women at the same table—none of them having ever met before—discovered they all lived on the same street in the same city within several blocks of each other! They all exchanged phone numbers and have become good friends. This happens a lot, in fact, and I want it to happen more without me having to travel to you to make it so. You can do this for yourself and other women in your community!

QUESTIONS FOR CARE PROVIDERS
AND BIRTH PLAN TEMPLATES

The following are some great questions to ask when interviewing care providers:

- Are you planning to be in town around my due date?
- What is my certainty that you or your backup will be available for my labor?
- If your backup isn't available to attend my birth, what's the plan?
- Who else will be assisting you during my labor?
- What's your rate of cesareans?
- Do you practice regular episiotomies—and if I say no, will I be listened to?
- What laboring options do you support—tub, birthing ball, etc.?
- How late will you support me past my baby's estimated due date—both legally and personally?
- How many weeks are you comfortable with me going past 40 weeks? What is the reasoning behind your answer?
- How often do you do cervical exams, and will you support my choice to decline them if I decide at any time to do so?
- Do you support a family-centered cesarean—a cesarean birth planned in such a way that the birthing person feels part of the birth experience and immediately postpartum, with options for things like skin-to-skin contact following surgery and dropping the curtain or sheet so I can see my baby being born? Even if you are not planning one, it's good to ask to learn more about what kind of provider they are, and so that you know your options if it does become a possibility or need.
- Do you have any questions for me?

If you're a VBAC birthing mama, you'll want to ask:

- Do you support a VBAC?
- What are your transfer rates (from home or birthing center to hospital)?
- How many of your transfers have vaginal births and how many have cesareans? Why?
- If I go past 40 weeks, how long are you comfortable waiting?
- What are my options before a repeat cesarean?
- Do you support different labor positions, other than lying on my back?

Other things you may start thinking about and discuss with your care provider:

- How do you and the hospital feel about delayed cord clamping?
- How do you and the hospital feel about skin-to-skin bonding?
- What are your and the hospital's policies on delayed hepatitis B vaccine, vitamin K, and silver nitrate?

HOSPITAL BIRTH PLAN TEMPLATE

Parent(s) Name(s):
Baby (boy/girl/surprise): [child's name]
Estimated Due Date:
Hospital: [location name]
Mother's Physician: [doctor's/midwife's name]
Doula:

I/We prefer the following during labor and delivery:

☐ A vaginal delivery over a cesarean.
☐ Membranes are not to be artificially ruptured.

- [ ] As few medications and/or medical interventions as necessary.
- [ ] Pain medication is not to be offered unless [mother's name] requests it.
- [ ] Saline lock (or hep-lock) to be used instead of a continuous IV.
- [ ] Freedom to move and choose position during labor and pushing stage.
- [ ] Use of intermittent fetal heart monitor (if continuous monitoring is *medically necessary*, a portable or wireless fetal heart monitor is preferred).
- [ ] Labor augmentation techniques are not to be used.
- [ ] No restrictions on [mother's name]'s urge to push.
- [ ] A local anesthetic to perineal area only if [mother's name] feels it is necessary.
- [ ] Risk tearing perineum instead of episiotomy.
- [ ] Natural delivery of the placenta.

I/We prefer the following immediately after delivery and postpartum:

- [ ] Skin-to-skin bonding with [child's name] immediately after birth.
- [ ] Initiation of breastfeeding as soon as possible after birth (if this is the mother's wish).
- [ ] Delayed clamping and cutting until umbilical cord has stopped pulsating.
- [ ] Allow [father's/partner's name] to cut the umbilical cord.
- [ ] Delayed newborn measurements, tests, and/or procedures until after sufficient skin-to-skin bonding and initial breastfeeding unless medical necessity dictates otherwise.
- [ ] No silver nitrate eye gel, vitamin K shot, or hepatitis B vaccine to be given to [child's name] immediately following birth without [mother's name]'s consent. If needed, [mother's name] will sign a waiver before surgery.

- [ ] [Child's name] is to be kept in room with [mother's name] at all times for the duration of hospital stay.
- [ ] All medical tests and/or procedures are to be done in room with [mother's name] and/or [father's/partner's name] present at *all* times.
- [ ] If [child's name] must go to the NICU due to medical necessity, [father's/partner's name] will be accompanying.
- [ ] If visitors arrive, please consult with [mother's name] and/or [father's/partner's name] before allowing them in the room.
- [ ] No pacifiers, artificial nipples, bottles, formula, or water are to be given to [child's name] for the duration of the hospital stay without [mother's name]'s and/or [father's/partner's name]'s consent.

CESAREAN BIRTH PLAN TEMPLATE

Parent(s) Name(s):
Baby (boy/girl/surprise): [child's name]
Estimated Due Date:
Hospital: [location name]
Mother's Physician: [doctor's name]
- [ ] Only use medications suitable for breastfeeding.
- [ ] If possible, provide a non-drowsy, anti-nausea medication.
- [ ] Explain the surgery to [mother's name] as it is being performed.
- [ ] Provide a warm blanket during the surgery.
- [ ] Provide a clear screen so [mother's name] may view the birth. If a clear screen is not possible, lower the screen just before the delivery so [mother's name] may view the birth.
- [ ] Perform surgery slowly enough to allow baby to breathe on his or her own while the umbilical cord continues to pulsate.

I/We prefer the following immediately after delivery and in recovery:

☐ No sedatives are to be given after the birth so [mother's name] can be alert and attentive during [child's name]'s first day of life.

☐ Double-suture the uterus with dissolvable stitches and suture external layers instead of using staples.

☐ Facilitate skin-to-skin bonding with [child's name] immediately after birth. If not possible, [father's/partner's name] will bond skin-to-skin with the baby.

☐ Initiate breastfeeding as soon as possible after birth unless medical necessity dictates otherwise (if this is the mother's wish).

☐ Allow [father's/partner's name] to cut the umbilical cord.

☐ Newborn measurements, tests, and/or procedures are to be delayed until after sufficient skin-to-skin bonding and initial breastfeeding, unless medical necessity dictates otherwise.

☐ No silver nitrate eye gel, vitamin K shot, or hepatitis B vaccine is to be given to [child's name] immediately following birth without [mother's name]'s consent. If needed, [mother's name] will sign a waiver before surgery.

☐ When [mother's name] has been cleared as stable and taken to a recovery room, she and [father's/partner's name] would like to be left alone to breastfeed [child's name] in a peaceful environment.

☐ [Mother's name] would like a snack or meal and to have IV removed as soon as possible following surgery.

☐ [Mother's name] will be nursing [child's name] often in order to stimulate production of breastmilk and soothe baby.

☐ [Child's name] is to be kept in room with [mother's name] at all times for the duration of the hospital stay.

☐ All medical tests and/or procedures are to be done in room with [mother's name] and/or [father's/partner's name] present at *all* times.

- ☐ [Child's name]'s bath is to be delayed until the evening following birth.
- ☐ If [child's name] must go to the NICU (neonatal intensive care unit) due to medical necessity, [father's/partner's name] will be accompanying.
- ☐ Remove [mother's name]'s catheter the evening or morning after surgery.
- ☐ [Mother's name] will be up and walking as soon as possible.
- ☐ If visitors arrive, please consult with [mother's name] and/or [father's/partner's name] before allowing them in the room.
- ☐ No pacifiers, artificial nipples, bottles, formula, or water are to be given to [child's name] for the duration of the hospital stay without [mother's name]'s and/or [father's/partner's name]'s consent.

HOME BIRTH PLAN TEMPLATE

Parent(s) Name(s):

Baby (boy/girl/surprise): [child's name]

Estimated Due Date:

Midwife (Team, if applicable): [midwife's name, assistant midwife's name]

Doula: [doula's name]

Other Support People: [birth photographer, friends, family, caregiver for siblings]

I/We prefer the following during labor and birth:

- ☐ Environment to be regulated according to [mother's name]'s preferences, such as conversations and noises kept to a minimum, lights dimmed or off, specific music or playlist to be played, water kept to a comfortable temperature range in birthing tub (if applicable), specific essential oils to be diffused, etc.

☐ No mention or discussion of time unless [mother's name] asks.

☐ To be left alone with [father's/partner's name] when requested.

☐ Cervical checks kept to a minimum and done only when deemed medically necessary by [midwife's name] and consented to by [mother's name].

☐ [Mother's name] is GBS-positive and [consents/does not consent] to chlorhexidine wash during labor.

☐ [Mother's name] is GBS-positive and [consents/does not consent] to antibiotics (at early labor/when water breaks).

☐ Use of (Doppler/fetoscope) for intermittent fetal monitoring.

☐ Monitoring of [mother's name]'s vitals to be kept to a minimum unless [midwife's name] deems it medically necessary.

☐ Recommendations to ease labor, such as breathing techniques, pain relief, hot and/or cold compresses, etc.

☐ Healthy snack suggestions and reminders to stay hydrated to maintain [mother's name]'s energy.

☐ Frequent checking in and encouragement during labor.

☐ Freedom to move and choose position during labor and pushing stage.

☐ Suggestions and/or help to guide pushing if needed.

☐ [Midwife's name] to [give/not give] perineal support and/or massage during labor.

☐ [Mother's name] or [father's/partner's name] to catch the baby if requested.

☐ Birth photographer to be present to take pictures (if applicable).

☐ No one else present during labor without [mother's name]'s consent.

I/We prefer the following immediately after birth and postpartum:

- ☐ Skin-to-skin bonding with [child's name] immediately after birth.
- ☐ [Mother's name] or [husband/partner's name] to announce the gender if it's unknown.
- ☐ Initiation of breastfeeding as soon as possible after birth (if this is the mother's wish).
- ☐ Natural delivery of the placenta, no managed third stage of labor or cord traction, unless intervention is medically necessary for safety of [mother's name].
- ☐ Delayed clamping and cutting until umbilical cord has stopped pulsating.
- ☐ Allow [father's/partner's name] to cut the umbilical cord or cord burning if preferred.
- ☐ Delayed newborn measurements and tests until after sufficient skin-to-skin bonding and initial breastfeeding, unless medical necessity dictates otherwise.
- ☐ No silver nitrate eye gel or vitamin K shot to be given to [child's name] immediately following birth without [mother's name]'s consent. Discuss delay or alternatives.
- ☐ [Child's name] is to be kept with [mother's name] at all times.

Note: If a hospital transfer is necessary, please refer to the hospital birth plan. If a C-section is needed after transferring to the hospital, please refer to the cesarean birth plan.

BIRTHING CENTER BIRTH PLAN TEMPLATE

Parent(s) Name(s):
Baby (boy/girl/surprise): [child's name]

Estimated Due Date:

Birthing Center: [location name]

Mother's Midwife: [midwife's name]

Doula:

I/We prefer the following during labor and delivery:

☐ Membranes are not to be artificially ruptured.

☐ As few medications and/or medical interventions as necessary.

☐ Pain medication is not to be offered unless [mother's name] requests it.

☐ Saline lock (or hep-lock) to be used instead of a continuous IV, if an IV is deemed medically necessary.

☐ Freedom to move and choose position during labor and pushing stage.

☐ Use of intermittent fetal heart monitor (if continuous monitoring is *medically necessary*, a portable or wireless fetal heart monitor is preferred).

☐ Labor augmentation techniques are not to be used.

☐ No restrictions on [mother's name]'s urge to push.

☐ A local anesthetic to perineal area only if [mother's name] feels it is necessary.

☐ Risk tearing perineum instead of episiotomy.

☐ Natural delivery of the placenta.

I/We prefer the following immediately after delivery and postpartum:

☐ Skin-to-skin bonding with [child's name] immediately after birth.

☐ Initiation of breastfeeding as soon as possible after birth (if this is the mother's wish).

☐ Clamping and cutting umbilical cord delayed until it has stopped pulsating.

- [ ] Allow [father's/partner's name] to cut the umbilical cord.
- [ ] Newborn measurements, tests, and/or procedures to be delayed until after sufficient skin-to-skin bonding and initial breastfeeding, unless medical necessity dictates otherwise.
- [ ] No silver nitrate eye gel or vitamin K shot to be given to [child's name] immediately following birth without [mother's name]'s consent. If needed, [mother's name] will sign the waiver before the surgery.
- [ ] [Child's name] is to be kept in room with [mother's name] at all times for the duration of hospital stay.
- [ ] All medical tests and/or procedures are to be done in room with [mother's name] and/or [father's/partner's name] present at *all* times.
- [ ] If visitors arrive, please consult with [mother's name] and/or [father's/partner's name] before allowing them in the room.
- [ ] No pacifiers, artificial nipples, bottles, formula, or water are to be given to [child's name] for the duration of the hospital stay without [mother's name]'s and/or [father's/partner's name]'s consent.

Glossary

Baby-friendly hospital: a hospital accredited by the Baby Friendly Hospital Initiative (BFHI), a global program launched by the World Health Organization and UNICEF in 1991 to protect, promote, and support breastfeeding. A hospital designated as "baby friendly" has been inspected and meets strict criteria centered on enabling new mothers to breastfeed for the first six months of their newborn's life.

Babywearing: the practice of carrying a baby or toddler close to your body in a baby carrier or sling while involved in day-to-day activities.

Back labor: intense lower back pain that peaks during contractions. This can be affected by the position of the baby.

Birthing center: a health care facility specifically centered on childbirth where midwives attend to expectant and laboring mothers. Birthing centers tend to enable laboring women to make informed choices on their care, often serving as a happy medium between a hospital birth and a home birth.

Birth philosophy: your thoughts, ideas, and views regarding labor and birth.

Birth pool: a tub used by an expectant mother to labor and/or birth her baby. Birth pools for home births are most often portable and/or inflatable. Most birthing centers have birth pools of their own for laboring and birthing women to use.

Birth team: the care and support group you choose to surround yourself with during labor and baby's birth, consisting of your care provider(s), partner, family, friend(s), doula(s), etc.

Breast pump: a mechanical device used to extract milk from the breasts of a lactating woman. Breast pumps can be electrical, battery operated, or manually operated (handheld).

Breech presentation: when the baby is in a bottom-first or feet-first position inside the womb.

- **Complete breech:** bottom first with both arms and both legs flexed in a fetal position.
- **Footling breech:** one foot or both feet up by the baby's head, sometimes exiting the birth canal first.
- **Frank breech:** bottom first with both legs extended up by the baby's head.
- **Incomplete breech:** bottom first with both arms and one leg flexed while the other leg is extended up by the baby's head.

CBAC: cesarean birth after a cesarean.

Cervical exam: similar to the pelvic exam for non-pregnant women, but with more attention given to the cervix and its indication as to whether labor has begun or is progressing.

Cervix: the narrow lower end of the uterus that the baby passes through during childbirth.

Childbirth education class: a class taught by a trained childbirth educator, consisting of lectures, discussions, and exercises aimed at preparing the pregnant woman (and her partner) for childbirth. Some common examples are Lamaze, the Bradley method, and hypnobirthing. Classes may vary widely based on type of class taught, teacher, and location.

Contraction (or uterine contraction): the tightening and shortening of the uterus that causes the cervix to thin and dilate, as well as aid the baby's descent into the birth canal.

Cytotec: a drug used to induce labor by softening the cervix. Taken by mouth or as a suppository. The FDA warns against its use by pregnant women due to possible abortion. Informed consent is a must.

Diastasis recti: separation between the abdominal muscles that can occur after pregnancy. Sometimes it may heal on its own; sometimes this needs greater attention from a care provider, such as a physical therapist or your medical doctor.

Directed pushing (or purple pushing): when the care provider requires the laboring woman to take a deep breath, hold it for a count of ten, and then push as hard as possible, whether she feels the urge to push or not. The woman's face will turn red or purple, eyes can begin to bulge, and blood vessels in the eyes may burst.

Doula: a person trained to assist and support a birthing woman and who may also provide additional support to the family after the birth.

Due date: the estimated date of your baby's birth. Due dates are typically calculated by adding 40 weeks to the first day of your last menstrual period (28-day cycle). If your baby is born on the due date, he or she is actually 38 weeks if you take into account the menstrual period and ovulation as the first two weeks of pregnancy.

Epidural: continuous pain relief for the lower half of the body during labor. Medication is administered through a catheter into the epidural space outside the membrane surrounding your spinal cord and spinal fluid.

Episiotomy: a surgical incision of the perineum to enlarge the vaginal opening for the baby to pass through. Done by an obstetrician or midwife during the second stage of labor if fetal distress is present. Informed consent is an absolute must.

Face presentation: when the baby is positioned head down, but presents face-first due to extension of the neck, as if the baby is in a "looking up" position.

Family-centered cesarean (or gentle cesarean): the act of creating a calm and peaceful atmosphere around a cesarean birth, where the birthing person feels part of the birth experience and immediately after in such a way that it closely resembles how a vaginal childbirth and postpartum would have been planned out.

Fetal heart rate monitoring: checking on the baby's condition by their heart rate through auscultation or electronic fetal monitoring.

- **Auscultation:** periodically listening to the fetal heartbeat through the use of a special stethoscope or a fetal Doppler.
- **Electronic fetal monitoring:** continuous recording of the fetal heartbeat in response to the laboring woman's contractions with an electronic fetal monitor. Can be external or internal.

First trimester: the first twelve weeks of pregnancy.

Fourth trimester: a term used for the first twelve weeks of postpartum following childbirth.

Gas and air (or laughing gas): a colorless, odorless gas used to take the edge off labor and any pain associated with labor.

HBAC: home birth after a cesarean.

Inducing labor: the intentional act of starting or increasing the speed of labor under medical supervision using interventions such as herbs, Pitocin, membrane sweep, foley bulb, etc. Informed consent is a must.

Infertility: the inability to get pregnant due to an inadequate level of specific hormones in one or both partners.

- **Secondary infertility:** the inability to get pregnant or carry a pregnancy full term after having one child. Causes may be attributed to (but are not limited to) uterine adhesions after a cesarean or scarring due to a uterus infection or retained placenta.

Informed consent: permission given to the health care provider to proceed with treatment after the patient has first been informed of all possible risks and benefits.

Intervention: when your care provider intervenes for health and safety reasons. Common interventions are electronic fetal monitoring, methods to induce labor, directed pushing, episiotomy, and cesarean. Informed consent is a must.

Labor: the process by which your body begins to prepare itself to birth a baby. It is divided into three stages:

- **First stage:** starts when contractions begin and ends when cervix dilates. Divided into two phases:
    1. **Early labor:** when your cervix effaces and dilates.
    2. **Active labor:** when the cervix dilates more frequently. Contractions become longer, more intense, and more frequent. The final part of active labor is referred to as transition.
- **Second stage:** also referred to as the pushing stage. Starts when the cervix is fully dilated and ends when the baby is born.
- **Third stage:** starts immediately after the birth of the baby and ends with the delivery of the placenta.

Labor positions: favorable positions in which the birthing person feels most comfortable.

- **Birthing bar:** can be attached to hospital labor beds to allow for a supported squatting position.
- **Birth stool:** a stool to sit in a low squat position to help open the pelvis.
- **Kneeling while draped over a bed or birth ball:** may be effective for reducing back labor.
- **Side-lying:** allows for rest between pushing contractions.
- **Sitting upright:** a variation of the position used on the birth stool.
- **Squatting:** the squat expands the pelvis and aids in the baby's descent into the birth canal.

Lactation: the secretion of breastmilk by the mammary glands.

Lactation consultant: a breastfeeding specialist trained to instruct and support mothers in feeding their new baby. Lactation consultants can help overcome issues that arise during breastfeeding, such as difficulty with latching on, painful nursing, and low milk production. Sometimes called an IBCLC, short for International Board Certified Lactation Consultant.

Membrane sweep (or stripping membranes): when the care provider inserts his or her finger into the cervix to separate the bag of water from the uterine wall to induce labor. Informed consent is a must.

Midwife: a person trained as a specialist to look after a pregnant woman throughout her entire pregnancy, childbirth, and postpartum care.

- **Certified midwife (CM):** has completed a graduate-level midwife program accredited by the Accreditation Commission for Midwifery Education (ACME) and passed the certification exam administered by the American Midwifery Certification Board.
- **Certified nurse-midwife (CNM):** a registered nurse who has completed a graduate-level nurse-midwife program accredited by ACME and passed the certification exam administered by the American Midwifery Certification Board.
- **Certified professional midwife (CPM):** has met the certification requirements of the North American Registry of Midwives (NARM) by serving as an apprentice to a certified midwife or graduating from an accredited midwifery school or program, both of which require completing the entry-level portfolio evaluation process.
- **Lay midwife (LM):** an uncertified or unlicensed midwife, usually consisting of an apprenticeship or self-study. Some states require licensing for lay midwives.

Midwifery care: care by a midwife that includes overseeing the well-being of the mother and her baby over the course of pregnancy, birth, and postpartum.

NICU: neonatal intensive care unit. Specializes in caring for premature or sick newborn babies.

OB/GYN: a medical doctor specializing in obstetrics and gynecology.

Oxytocin: hormone secreted by the pituitary gland and known as the "cuddle hormone" or "love hormone" due to its release during physical bonding, such as hugging or cuddling. It also strengthens labor contractions and helps stabilize bleeding after childbirth. Artificial oxytocin is used in hospitals to induce labor under the brand name Pitocin.

Perineum: the space between the anus and vulva.

Pitocin: brand name for artificial oxytocin. Administered intravenously to induce labor. Informed consent is a must.

Placenta: the organ that develops inside the uterus during pregnancy and is attached to the growing baby within by the umbilical cord.

- **Anterior placenta:** when the placenta is attached to the front wall of the uterus. May result in difficulty feeling the baby move.
- **Placenta previa (or low-lying placenta):** when the placenta partially or completely covers the cervix. Severe bleeding may be a symptom before and/or during labor. Frequent or intermittent bleeding is possible during the second half of the pregnancy.
- **Posterior placenta:** when the placenta is attached to the back wall of the uterus.

Postdates: when the pregnancy goes more than two weeks beyond the given due date.

Postpartum (PP): any time after the baby is born.

Postpartum depression (PPD): depression occurring after and possibly as a result of childbirth.

Post-Traumatic Stress Disorder (PTSD): a disorder resulting from witnessing or experiencing a frightening event.

Prenatal depression (or antenatal depression): depression occurring during pregnancy.

Ring of fire: the burning sensation felt when the labia and perineum are stretched to the maximum during childbirth.

Rooming in: when the newborn baby is kept in the same room as the mother to allow for better bonding in the postpartum period immediately following childbirth.

Round ligament pain: may occur during the second trimester as your belly grows. Sensation or discomfort as the ligament in your lower belly or groin area stretches and expands.

Second trimester: week 13 through week 27 of pregnancy.

Shoulder presentation: when the baby is sideways inside the womb and the shoulder or arm enter the birth canal first. Usually cause for a cesarean.

Skin-to-skin: the act of bonding between the new mother and newborn baby immediately after the birth by placing the naked baby on the mother's bare chest. If not possible for the mother, then the father, spouse, partner, etc. may step in.

Swaddling: the act of snugly wrapping the baby in a blanket to soothe and comfort him or her. Mimics the womb by restricting movement of the limbs, and helps the baby feel safe and secure and sleep better.

TENS unit: TENS stands for transcutaneous electrical nerve stimulation. A device that sends a stimulating electrical current across the skin and nerves to block pain signals from reaching the brain, as well as produce higher levels of endorphins, your body's own natural painkillers.

Third trimester: week 28 of pregnancy until birth.

Transferred care: when transfer of prenatal care from one OB or midwife to another is necessary due to risk, complications during labor, or differing opinions with current provider during pregnancy.

* **in pregnancy:** refers to switching of care providers.
* **in labor:** refers to hospital transfer under the care of an OB due to complications or differing opinions during labor at a birthing center or at home under the care of a midwife.

Transition: the final stage of active labor.

Trial of labor (TOL): labor under the supervision of an OB, usually with restrictions and limits.

Uterus: also known as the womb. The hollow muscular organ in the female pelvis where the baby and placenta develop. The narrow lower end that opens up is the cervix.

VBAC: vaginal birth after a cesarean.

VBAC-friendly provider: an OB or midwife comfortable with overseeing a mother's attempt at having a vaginal birth after a previous cesarean birth.

VBA2C: vaginal birth after two cesareans.

WIC (Women, Infants, and Children): WIC programs provide supplemental foods, health care referrals, and nutrition education for low-income pregnant, breastfeeding, and non-breastfeeding postpartum women, and to infants and children up to age five.

Notes

1. Marlena S. Fejzo PhD, Kimber W. MacGibbon RN, Roberto Romero MD, T. Murphy Goodwin MD, Patrick M. Mullin MD, "Recurrence Risk of Hyperemesis Gravidarum," *Journal of Midwifery and Women's Health* 52, no. 2 (March 2011): 132.
2. "Miscarriage," *March of Dimes*, November 2017, accessed at https://www.marchofdimes.org/complications/miscarriage.aspx.
3. Melissa Bruijn and Debby Gould, "The Pitfalls of 'Going with the Flow' in Birth," March 26, 2012. Accessed June 20, 2017, at https://birthtraumatruths.wordpress.com/2012/03/26/the-pitfalls-of-going-with-the-flow-in-birth/.
4. Recent scientific research on health and obesity increasingly questions the link between being overweight and being unhealthy. See Jason Hu, "The Obesity Paradox," *Quartz*, November 17, 2015. Accessed July 28, 2017, at https://qz.com/550527/obesity-paradox-scientists-now-think-that-being-overweight-is-sometimes-good-for-your-health/.
5. See "Definition of Term Pregnancy," Committee Opinion No. 579, American College of Obstetricians and Gynecologists, *Obstetrics and Gynecology* 122, no. 5 (November 2013): 1139–40.
6. The Baby-Friendly Hospital Initiative is developed and implemented by UNICEF and the World Health Organization, which work with national authorities across many countries. Baby-Friendly USA is the accrediting organization for the United States. Accessed at https://www.babyfriendlyusa.org.
7. Joyce A. Martin, MPH; Brady E. Hamilton, PhD; Michelle J. K. Osterman, MHS.; Anne K. Driscoll, PhD; and T. J. Mathews, MS, "Births: Final Data for 2015," *National Vital Statistics Report* 66, no. 1, p. 2, accessed at https://www.cdc.gov/nchs/fastats/delivery.htm.
8. Ana Pilar Betran; Jianfeng Ye; Anne-Beth Moller; Jun Zhang; A. Metin Gulmezoglu; and Maria Regina Torloni, "The Increasing Trend in Ceasarean Section Rates: Global, Regional and National Estimates: 1990–2014," *Plos*

One, February 5, 2016, accessed December 8, 2017 at https://www.ncbi.nlm
.nih.gov/pmc/articles/PMC4743929/.

9. *Health at a Glance 2015: OECD Indicators*, OECD Publishing, Paris, p.
115; and World Health Organization, "Caesarean Sections Should Only
Be Performed When Medically Necessary," news release, April 10, 2015,
accessed December 8, 2017 at http://www.who.int/mediacentre/news/
releases/2015/caesarean-sections/en/.

10. "Birthing Choices: Health Care and Providers and Birth Locations," *American Pregnancy Association*, September 2016, accessed December 8, 2017 at
http://americanpregnancy.org/labor-and-birth/birthing-choices/.

11. Amely Greeven, "One Writer's Journey from Skinny to Strong," *W Magazine*, February 20, 2017, accessed December 8, 2017 at https://www.wmagazine
.com/story/building-muscle-strong-body-journey.

12. See this article in *Parents Magazine*, for example: http://www.parents.com/
parenting/dads/101/health-benefits-of-fatherhood/. See also this study from
the Pew Research Center: http://www.pewresearch.org/fact-tank/2017/06/15/
fathers-day-facts/.

Recommended Resources

If you love the idea of a harmony circle but not the idea of organizing one (I get it—sometimes it's just the last thing you want to do), I want to help you create that support system in other ways. Here are some of my favorite books, websites, social media accounts, and organizations that align with the Birth Without Fear philosophy for options, support, and respect, self-care, and self-love.

Pursue what speaks to you here. I know there have been times in my pregnancy and postpartum journeys when a Snapchat postpartum buddy, a breastfeeding support group's hotline, or a blog post have quite literally saved my life. It doesn't have to be all or nothing—a combination of community gathering, deep dives into book or blog reading, or shorter bursts of support with Instagram posts or Facebook group questions can all make a difference in their own ways as needed or wanted.

I can't promise that all of these resources will have the same "no judgment, just love" philosophy as Birth Without Fear, so please take or leave them as needed and helpful—and approach with the same focus on options, support, and respect that I've encouraged you to approach everything with all along!

Books I Read to Prepare for My Births

Pam England, CNM, MA, and Rob Horowitz, PhD. *Birthing from Within: An Extra-Ordinary Guide to Childbirth Preparation*. Albuquerque: Partera Press, 1998.

Marie F. Mongon, M.Ed., M.Hy., *HypnoBirthing, Fourth Edition: A Natural Approach to Safer, Easier, More Comfortable Birthing—The Mongon Method.* Deerfield Beach: Health Communications, Inc., 2015.

Peggy Vincent. *Baby Catcher: Chronicles of a Modern Midwife.* New York: Scribner, 2003.

Books Also Loved by the Birth Without Fear Community

The Birth Partner by Penny Simkin.
Birth with Confidence by Rhea Dempsey.
Gentle Birth, Gentle Mothering by Sarah J Buckley.
Supernatural Childbirth by Jackie Mize.
The Thinking Woman's Guide to a Better Birth by Henci Goer.
The Womanly Art of Breastfeeding by La Leche League International.
Also: *The Business of Being Born*, documentary by Ricki Lake and Abby Epstein.

Additional Websites, Organizations, and Support

Birth Without Fear is the most obvious choice, of course! You will get the most comprehensive information, support, and validation you can get as a pregnant woman, birthing person, or new mom by visiting Birth Without Fear at the following locations:
birthwithoutfearblog.com
facebook.com/birthwithoutfear
instagram.com/birthwithoutfear

For new moms going through the exhausting journey of postpartum and struggling with self-love, body positivity, and self-care, please visit Take Back Postpartum on Instagram:
instagram.com/takebackpostpartum

If you enjoyed the Partner Point of View sections in this book, you can get even more by visiting Don't Forget Dads on Instagram:
   instagram.com/dontforgetdads

If you are interested in attending a live Birth Without Fear Conference where you will be loved, supported, validated, and uplifted, please go to our event website and register for an event near you at:
   bwfconference.com

If you want to hear Brandon and me discuss everything from birth and parenting to coffee and marriage, you can listen to *The Harshē Podcast* at:
   harshe.blog/podcast

If you love birth stories, Bryn Huntpalmer hosts *The Birth Hour* podcast where she interviews women from all walks of life about their own unique birth experiences at:
   thebirthhour.com

Some other websites of note are:
   International Cesarean Awareness Network (ICAN):
      ican-online.org
   La Leche League International: dev.llli.org
   Fearless Formula Feeder: fearlessformulafeeder.com
   Mocha Moms: mochamoms.org
   Black Women Do Breastfeed: blackwomendobreastfeed.org
   Black Women Birthing Justice: blackwomenbirthingjustice.org
   National Center for Fathering: fathers.com

The following are safe and confidential resources for when you need support *right now*. Sometimes we truly need to feel that we are not alone for a moment, and these organizations can and will provide that space for you. Please use them if you need or want to. They are there for you. We added the websites for you to research them further if you are not quite comfortable talking to someone yet. It's scary opening ourselves up, feeling vulnerable, and fearing the outcome of doing so. Those are real, valid, and common feelings. These organizations know that and work hard to ease those fears, to simply hold space and be there for you. I know I cannot hold your hand and listen to you over a cup of coffee, although I wish I could, so this is what I can do instead: hold your hand in theory, give you information, and encourage you to get the support you deserve. You are amazing and needed and wanted and loved. You are enough. You are worthy.

Postpartum Support International: postpartum.net or
1-800-944-4773

Suicide Prevention Lifeline: suicidepreventionlifeline.org or
1-800-273-TALK

Self Harm Hotline | One Love All Equal: oneloveallequal.org or 1-800-366-8288

Addiction | SAMHSA: samhsa.gov or 1-800-662-4357

National Eating Disorders Association: nationaleatingdisorders.org or 1-800-931-2237

National Domestic Violence Hotline: thehotline.org or
1-800-799-SAFE

Sexual Abuse Hotline: rainn.org or 1-800-656-HOPE

And please make, refer to, and use your own personal list that is unique to you: your local groups, therapist, midwife, OB, friend, neighbor, etc. If you don't have one, start making one. Research groups, support, therapists, and doctors in your community. They are there for you. If you find one who doesn't have your best interests at heart, move on until you find one that does. You would do it for your child, so do it for yourself. You are just as worthy and deserving.

Acknowledgments

These acknowledgments wouldn't feel right if I didn't start them by thanking the two women most responsible for this book being a reality.

One day in January 2017, I went through one of my many email inboxes and found a random email from November 2016 that I had simply missed—not an uncommon occurrence. It was from Colleen Martell. The email mentioned that she had followed me and Birth Without Fear for some time, that she worked for a book agent, and asked if I ever thought of writing a book. I replied that I had, but that I had been waiting for the right time and opportunity to take on such a project. When the thought of writing a book actually became a reality, Colleen helped me transfer my message of empowerment, solidarity, and love that I share all over social media and at Birth Without Fear events into the pages of a book as if I had just spoken them. Our Skype calls often turned into holding space for one another. We were practicing the words we so carefully wrote for all those who will read them. Colleen, there were many, many days that your passion for this book (and veganism!) inspired me and I can't imagine having done this without you.

A week after I responded to Colleen's first email, Brandon and I did a Skype call with Colleen and our soon-to-be book agent, Stephanie Tade. After the four of us talked and decided that we all wanted to make a Birth Without Fear book a reality, I broke down into tears of joy. In an hour's time, Stephanie validated the years of hard work and sleepless nights I put into Birth Without Fear, and she has continued to do so every single step of the way through this process—from guiding me through the subways of New York City to meet with numerous publishers, to the expectations I should have during the entire publishing process, to her advocacy of me and this book and what it will mean to women everywhere. I am so grateful for your wisdom and friendship, Stephanie, and I wouldn't want to do this with anyone but you. Let's do it again!

I next have to thank Michelle Howry for her belief in Birth Without Fear's potential as a book. Her positivity during the early stages of writing this book meant the world to me and I will never forget that.

Of course, I have to thank Lauren Hummel and the entire Hachette team for the hard work they've put into this book. Lauren has been a valuable guide during the publication process and her excitement is so palpable and fun! The support everyone at Hachette has shown for Birth Without Fear has been such a huge source of inspiration for me and has, quite honestly, gotten me through some very tough days. My gratitude for all of you is beyond words.

I also have to thank Julie Will and Karen Rinaldi at Harper Wave, Julia Pastore at HarperOne, Marian Lizzi at TarcherPerigree, Cara Bedick at Touchstone, and Renee Sedliar at Da Capo for all believing in this book as well. All of you helped me to know the true worth of Birth Without Fear.

To the hundreds of thousands of people who have followed Birth Without Fear online and on social media, you are the ones who started the momentum for a Birth Without Fear book. To the thousands who have attended a Birth Without Fear Conference or MeetUp or a Find Your Village gathering, you have shown me that Birth Without Fear's message is not only needed, it is necessary in changing the conversation we have about birth in the Western world. This book is literally for all of you. This is *our* voice.

To my grandparents, Joseph and JoAnn Callaway a.k.a. Nanny and Papa, thank you just doesn't seem like enough. You two have been in my corner from the moment of *my own birth* and have saved my life so many times I can't count them all. I love you both so much and I'm grateful and excited you are on this journey with me.

To my best friend and husband, Brandon, who's recommendation of what I should say of him (while hilarious) is not appropriate for this book, you are my partner and no one else knows, accepts, and loves me the way you do. You are my biggest champion and I am your biggest cheerleader. I love you a bunches of munches.

And most of all to my six babies. If someone would have told me years ago that all of your births would be massive learning experiences and the basis for writing a book one day, I would not have believed them. But they would have been right. I love you all so, so much and never could have done this without all of you in my life. You have each reminded me time and again of my own power and potential. You are a self-love generation and I am a better human being because of all of you.

Index

of postpartum sex and intimacy,
201–202, 204–205
in third trimester, 41–42
North American Registry of
Midwives (NARM), 114
Norway, 75
nuchal test, 22
nurses
certified nurse-midwives, 32, 108,
114, 236
labor and delivery, 62–63

OB/GYNs, 32–33, 48–49, 236
obsessive-compulsive disorder
(OCD), postpartum, 188
overweight individuals, 241n.4
oxytocin, 84, 208, 237

pain
with postpartum sex, 204, 205
round ligament, 23, 29, 238
pain management, 64, 103–104,
108–109
panic attacks, 3–4
parenthood, 131–134
parent(s)
expectations of, 163–165, 213–214
expectations placed on, 135–137
as members of birth team, 217–218
partner's role as, 153–154
self-care for, 138–141
partners and spouses
on birth team, 29, 30
during cesarean birth, 84–86
communication with, 202–204
encouragement of self-love by,
166–167
expectations about sex from,
205–206

feeding by, 179
fostering of confidence by, 94–96
home birth experience for, 117–119
mental health issues for, 195–197
parental role of, 153–154
participation in feeding by,
182–185
perspective of, on making backup
plans, 125–127
receipt of pregnancy news by,
18–20
reconnecting with, 199–202,
205–206
in second trimester, 36–38
self-care for, 151
self-confidence of, 52–54
support for, xviii, 36–38
support from, 20, 36–38, 84–86,
94–96
view of sex and intimacy by,
209–211
voice of, in hospital birth, 70–72
pediatrician, 59–60, 102
pelvic floor issues, 208–209
perinatal depression, 24–25
perineum, 237
pets, home birth and, 105
physical health, prioritization of,
22–23
Pitocin, 102, 237
placenta, 24, 237
placenta previa (low-lying placenta),
237
planned cesarean births, 77
plus-size moms, 26–28
PMS, symptoms of pregnancy vs., 5
pools, birth, 231
post-traumatic stress disorder
(PTSD), 90, 188, 193, 216, 237

About the Author

The mother of six amazing kids, January knows firsthand how widely birth experiences can vary, as she's run the gamut from an affirming and joyful planned cesarean to a traumatic emergency cesarean, as well as a VBA2C (vaginal birth after two cesareans) in the hospital, and two home births. One of these home births was such a dramatic departure from the confusion, uncertainty, and fear of her other births that a beautiful idea was born—she would make it her life's mission to promote a revolutionary birth and parenting message: you *can* have a birth without fear, no matter how you birth. In 2010 January founded the Birth Without Fear Facebook page and *Birth Without Fear* blog in order to spread her message of empowerment, to give women their voices back in the face of a powerful medical-industrial complex and widespread cultural ignorance about birth.

Soon, Birth Without Fear became so much more than a website—January had sparked a movement of information, inclusivity, and support. Her community had grown so big that January expanded her ventures so she could speak directly to areas of specific need. She created Take Back Postpartum, Don't Forget Dads, Breastfeed Without Fear, Find Your Village, and Raising Kids Without Fear, among others under the Birth Without Fear social media tent, which today represents a following of over one million and counting.

In 2013 January took Birth Without Fear on the road. She started with a wildly successful Birth Without Fear Conference in

Arlington, Texas, and then quickly developed a nationwide tour in 2014 to bring her message of information and empowerment to women across the United States. Since that first Birth Without Fear Conference, January has held over 100 events across North America and Australia.

January has been featured in the *Chicago Tribune*, *Huffington Post*, and *People*, as well as on ABC News. In those rare instances when she has a few free moments, January has been a regular contributing author to the *Huffington Post* since 2014. January also co-hosts *The Harshē Podcast* with her husband, Brandon, where they discuss everything related to kids, parenting, marriage, business, physical and mental health, tattoos, and coffee!

When January is not busy spreading her message of inspiration, solidarity, and body positivity to people everywhere, she enjoys eating tasty vegan food with Brandon, singing and dancing with her kids, drinking lots of coffee, and reading novels while soaking in a bath.

About the Author of Partner Point of View

As a chiropractor, Brandon Harshe is used to correcting problems, but nothing he learned in all those years of schooling and building a successful practice prepared him to support his partner or himself through pregnancy, birth, and parenting in today's culture. He needed to learn how to listen differently, find his own connection, and understand his own need for support and self-care. He needed to learn how to join in January's birth journeys without fear, and to trust his intuition as well as hers.

In 2015 Brandon joined January as a speaker at Birth Without Fear events, where he shares what he's learned as a father of six children and as January's central support person through pregnancies, loss, births, and postpartum. With hefty doses of humor and raw honesty, Brandon shares how powerless partners can feel during pregnancy and childbirth; when so much of the journey is beyond your control, when there's so much you can't fix, you need to learn other ways of being with your partner, he tells audiences. Oftentimes, the baby is the number-one concern for the mother, but until that baby is born, the mother is still the number-one concern for her partner—and this is such a meaningful, important role to play. It's hard and it's messy, he often confides, but he wants fathers and partners to know they aren't alone in their challenges. There is a way through if we can learn how to trust in her confidence in herself, and are open to new ways of connecting.

Brandon also helps run the *Birth Without Fear* blog, serving as webmaster and blog editor, and is highly involved in the decision-making process and evolution of Birth Without Fear and the Birth Without Fear events. He also co-hosts *The Harshē Podcast* with January, where he serves as the (sometimes inappropriate) comic relief. He once told January that millions of people were waiting to hear what she has to say. He was right. He's always in January's corner, unconditionally loving and supporting her as she supports others.

In his spare time, Brandon enjoys any time alone with January that he can get, watching superhero movies and shows with the kids, reading, writing, and playing the guitar.